Tal

TAKE CHARGE OF YOUR HEALTH

Healing with Yogatherapy and Nutrition

by Christopher S. Kilham

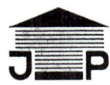

Japan Publications, Inc.

© 1985 by Christopher S. Kilham
Photographs by Mark Morrisroe

All rights reserved, including the right to reproduce this book or portions thereof in any form without the written permission of the publisher.

Note to the reader: The information contained in this book is not intended to be used in the diagnosis, prescription, or treatment of disease or any health disorder whatsoever. Nor is this information intended to replace competent medical care. This book is a compendium of information which may be used as an adjunct to a rational and responsible health care plan.

Published by JAPAN PUBLICATIONS, INC., Tokyo and New York

Distributors:
UNITED STATES: *Kodansha International/USA, Ltd., through Harper & Row, Publishers, Inc., 10 East 53rd Street, New York, New York 10022.* SOUTH AMERICA: *Harper & Row, Publishers, Inc., International Department.* CANADA: *Fitzhenry & Whiteside Ltd., 195 Allstate Parkway, Markham, Ontario L3R 4T8.* MEXICO AND CENTRAL AMERICA: *HARLA S. A de C. V., Apartado 30-546, Mexico 4, D. F.* BRITISH ISLES: *International Book Distributors Ltd., 66 Wood Lane End, Hemel Hempstead, Herts HP2 4RG.* EUROPEAN CONTINENT: *Fleetbooks, S. A., c/o Feffer and Simons (Nederland) B. V., Rijnkade 170, 1382 GT Weesp, The Netherlands.* AUSTRALIA AND NEW ZEALAND: *Bookwise International, 1 Jeanes Street, Beverley, South Australia 5007.* THE FAR EAST AND JAPAN: *Japan Publications Trading Co., Ltd., 1-2-1, Sarugaku-cho, Chiyoda-ku, Tokyo 101.*

First edition: October 1985

LCCC No. 84-082451
ISBN 0-87040-632-9

Printed in U.S.A.

*This book is lovingly dedicated to
Bette Day
my mother and friend.*

*Special thanks also to the former members
of the weekly Yoga classes
at the Boston Theosophical Society,
who for five years journeyed off dauntlessly
into the unknown, and found treasures there.*

Foreword

Over the past decade and a half, I have been pleased to observe and participate in a major social trend—the proliferation of self health care and natural healing modalities. It has become increasingly apparent that health care begins, not with the solicitation of a physician, but with awareness of, and interest in, the care and maintenance of one's own body and mind. Each of us has an opportunity to understand our health needs, and to learn how to take care of ourselves. To meet this opportunity with proficiency, we need information which will enable us to skillfully manage the daily operations of our well-being.

There is no definitive owner's manual for the Body/Mind. Instead, there are thousands of experts with thousands of opinions about how to stay healthy and vibrant. For every opinion or theory, there is opposition and challenge, as well as acceptance and support. In this curious world of ours, there may not actually be any ultimately true health system. Instead, it may be that information grows and evolves as we do, is useful and poignant one day, and is outdated later. With all of these considerations in mind, I offer *Take Charge of Your Health* as a timely compilation of health information which combines a variety of time-tested approaches to keeping oneself vibrant and well, without making exaggerated claims of eternal truth.

To learn about oneself is exciting and challenging. As far as I know, there is no end to that process. To take care of oneself can be satisfying and strengthening, imparting confidence and a sense of self-reliance. *Take Charge of Your Health* is full of information that can be used to prevent health disorders, and bring the Body/Mind back into balance if that balance has been upset. It is my wish for the reader that this volume will broaden your horizons, give you more choices, and contribute to your personal journey in a positive, generative way.

Being healthy is one aspect of a far greater process. I believe that we are here to enjoy ourselves, to be happy and delighted, and to unravel the mysteries of this awesome world. I hope that this book will assist you in staying healthy, so that you can happily pursue other, infinitely more exciting things.

CHRISTOPHER KILHAM
Northern California, 1984

Contents

Foreword 7
Take Charge of Your Health 15

Yoga and Yogatherapy 17

Yoga and Yogatherapy *19*
Yogatherapy Can Change Your Life *21*
The Mind/Body Relationship *22*
Yoga Philosophy *25*
Life and Energy *29*
The Aura *31*
The Chakras *32*
Chakra Chart *34*
Including Yogatherapy in Your Daily Plan *36*
Advice on the Practice *37*
When Yogatherapy Is Not Recommended *37*
Learning to Breathe *38*
Yoga Postures and Exercises *39*
    Soorya Namaskar—Salute to the Sun 39
    The Rejuvenation Series 42
    The Squat 48
    The Wide Squat 49
    Palm Pose 49
    One Legged Pose 50
    Neck Pose 50
    Triangle Pose 51
    Side Stretch 52
    Standing Leg Stretch 52
    Palm to Floor Pose 53
    Standing Back Stretch 53
    Forward Knee Pose 54
    Forward Knee Pose with Back Stretch 54
    Forward Knee/Palm Pose 55
    Pointing Pose 55
    Knee to Chest Pose 56
    Seminal Control Pose 56

Supine Knee to Chest Pose   57
Wind Eliminating Pose   57
Moving Knees to Chest Pose   58
Inverted Leg Pose   58
Celibate Pose   59
Supine Spinal Twist   60
Crotch Stretch   61
Pelvic Pose   62
Easy Pose   62
Rock Pose   63
Hero Pose   63
Cow Head Pose   64
Lion Pose   64
Lotus Pose   65
Lotus Spinal Stretch   65
Butterfly Pose   66
Leg Splits   66
Mahamudra #1 (The Great Yogic Seal)   67
Mahamudra #2   68
Mahamudra #3   68
Abdominal Tensor Pose   69
Inclined Spinal Twist   70
Spinal Twist   70
Fish Pose   71
Grasshopper Pose   72
Locust Pose   72
Boat Pose   73
Bow Pose   73
Cobra Pose   74
Peacock Pose   74
Bridge Pose   75
Camel Pose   76
Inclined Pose   76
Wheel Pose   77
Plow Pose   78
Reverse Seal   78
Shoulder Stand   79
Corpse Pose   80

Ingredients of Natural Living   81

Nature's Three Great Healers   83
Sunshine   83
Fresh Air   84
Pure Water   85

The Benefits of Walking *87*
Sleep *88*
Hot and Cold Showers *89*
Regularity in Schedule and Habits *90*

Nutrition 91

Diet and Yogatherapy *93*
   Vital Foods 93
   Fresh Vegetables and Fruits 94
   Fresh Juices 95
   Nuts and Seeds 95
   Dairy Products and Eggs 96
   Whole Grains 97
   Meats and Fish 98
   What to Avoid 99
   Guidelines for Eating 101
The Yogatherapy Cleansing Program *103*
   Cleansing Daily Schedule 104
Super Foods *106*
Fasting *111*
Juices, How to Prepare Them *113*
Juice/Ailment Chart *113*

Vitamins, Minerals, and Food Supplements 115

Vitamins, Minerals, and Food Supplements *117*
The RDA=Recommended Dietary Allowances *119*
   The RDA—What Are They? 119
   How Are the RDA Determined? 119
   Biochemical Individuality 120
   What Does This Mean? 121
The Nutrient Section *122*
   Vitamin A (Retinol) 124
   Vitamin B_1 (Thiamine) 125
   Vitamin B_2 (Riboflavin) 126
   Niacin 126
   Vitamin B_6 (Pyridoxine) 127
   Vitamin B_{12} (Cyanocobalamin) 127
   Pantothenic Acid 128
   PABA (Para-Amino-Benzoic Acid) 128
   Folic Acid (Folacin) 129
   Biotin 129
   Choline 130

Inositol 130
Vitamin C (Ascorbic Acid) 130
Vitamin D 131
Vitamin E 131
"Vitamin F" (Unsaturated Fatty Acid) 132
Vitamin K (Phylloquinone) 132
Vitamin P (Bioflavonoids, including citrus bioflavonoids, rutin, hesperidin) 133
Calcium 133
Magnesium 133
Phosphorous 134
Iodine 134
Iron 135
Copper 135
Zinc 136
Sodium 136
Potassium 136
Manganese 137
Selenium 137
Chromium 137
Nature—Vite Quick Reference Chart 138
Food Supplements 140

Herbology 145

Herbs, What They Are, What They Do 147
Preparation and Use of Herbs 147
Individual Herb Chart 148
Herbal Formula/Ailment Chart 153
Herbal Tea Bag/Ailment Chart 162
Special Herbal Extracts and Tablets 163

Yogatherapy Repertory 167

How to Use the Yogatherapy Repertory 169
Acne 170
Adenoids, Tonsils 171
Alcoholism, Drug Addiction 172
Allergies, Hay Fever 173
Anemia 174
Appetite (poor, lack of) 175
Arterial Disease 176

Arthritis, Gout, Rheumatism *177*
Back Pain *178*
Bladder Disorders *179*
Blood Pressure, High *179*
Blood Pressure, Low *180*
Bronchitis *181*
Cold Extremities *182*
Colds *183*
Colitis *184*
Constipation *185*
Cystitis *186*
Diabetes *187*
Diarrhea *188*
Dysentery *189*
Ear Trouble (congestion, infection) *190*
Eczema *191*
Eyes (dimming of vision) *192*
Fatigue *193*
Halitosis *194*
Headaches *195*
Heart Disease *195*
Hemmorrhoids *196*
Hernia *197*
Hypoglycemia *198*
Indigestion *199*
Influenza *200*
Insomnia *201*
Kidney Disorders *202*
Liver, Gallbladder Disorders *203*
Lungs, Asthma *204*
Male Impotence, Prostate Disorders *205*
Menopause *206*
Menstrual Disorders, PMS (cramping, edema, discomfort) *207*
Nervousness, Relaxation, Stress Management *208*
Obesity *209*
Pregnancy *210*
Pyorrhea *211*
Rejuvenation *211*
Sciatica *212*
Scoliosis *213*
Sinus Disorders *214*
Smoking—To Quit *215*
Spinal Flexibility *216*

14/Contents

    Stomach Disorders (cramping, nausea, acidity) *217*
    Thyroid Disorders *218*
    Vaginitis *219*
    Varicose Veins *220*

Meditation Practice 221

    References 227
    Index 229

Take Charge of Your Health—

Take Charge of Your Health? Why not? After all, if you don't do that, who will? Nobody else will. You alone are responsible for yourself, and for making sure that you get the most out of your own Body/Mind. How do you go about doing that? There's exercise, nutrition, meditation, vitamins, herbs, and many, many ways to contribute to health.

Take Charge of Your Health came about as the answer to a question that was asked of me for years. The question was "Why doesn't somebody put a lot of this health information into one, single book?" It is difficult and time consuming to chase around, finding one book here, one book there, each offering a few tidbits on health.

Take Charge of Your Health contains seven chapters:

1. Yoga and Yogatherapy,
2. Ingredients of Natural Living,
3. Nutrition,
4. Vitamins, Minerals, and Food Supplements,
5. Herbology,
6. Yogatherapy Repertory,
7. Meditation.

Each of these chapters may be used by itself. The chapter on Yoga and Yogatherapy, for example, describes a wide variety of Yoga postures and techniques, all photographically illustrated. Chapter 1 is really a Yoga book in and of itself, and can be used separately or in conjunction with the other chapters of the book.

The first five chapters of the book stand on their own, each offering a different kind of information. Chapter 6, the Yogatherapy Repertory, ties the various kinds of information together into 54 different programs for specific health conditions. Chapter 7 offers a complete description of a powerful meditation technique.

If you are in search of answers to personal health questions, or if you want to embark upon a personalized health program, the materials in this book will enable you to do exactly that. If, on the other hand, you are a health practitioner, you will find this book to be a useful reference for your own practice.

Whatever your personal reasons for reading this book, you will find a great deal of information that will help you to *Take Charge of Your Health!*

YOGA and YOGATHERAPY

Yoga and Yogatherapy

The vast systems of Yoga originate from India and the Northern regions of Nepal and Tibet, and are thousands of years old. From them is derived the classical Hindu science of *Ayurveda*, a detailed and effective health care system which plays a key role in Yogatherapy. *Ayurveda* is the primary health program of hundreds of millions of Asians, and its sophistication has not gone unnoticed by orthodox Western medical researchers.

Over the past few decades, the Western world has been exposed to many of the systems of Yoga. There are many components of the Yogic Way, including dietary practices, physical exercise, and meditation. Of these three broad categories of activity, there are literally thousands of methods for the attainment of radiant health, brilliant mental clarity, and spiritual fulfillment.

One of the most popular branches of Yoga is Hatha Yoga. This is a highly advanced system of physical postures, exercises, breathing techniques, concentration techniques, and meditation. These are combined with dietary disciplines, forming a solid program for total rejuvenation. Through regular practice of Hatha Yoga, one can positively revolutionize the health and vitality of the body and mind. Hatha Yoga is the most popular Yogic system among Westerners. Unless otherwise indicated, use of the word "Yoga" in this book will refer to the varied practices of Hatha Yoga.

The Yogic understanding is that life is in harmony when there is a balance of all the forces that make up a human being. As translated from the ancient Sanskrit language, the word Hatha means Sun/Moon, indicating a blend of cosmic forces. Hatha Yoga is a way to attain an exquisite balance of the forces in oneself. The practice is a way to experience the vibrant, joyfulness of life. Thus Hatha Yoga is a path of fulfillment.

Yogic practice is often thought to be exotic or difficult, and therefore out of reach for most people. Actually, the Yogic systems are all designed systematically to accommodate novices or experts. The practice of Hatha Yoga is readily available to anyone wanting to improve their health and vitality. Many of the Hatha Yoga techniques are well within the grasp of the beginner. Yet as with any endeavor worth pursuing, one must work persistently to become a Yoga adept.

Yoga postures and exercises tone and strengthen muscles, stretch and strengthen the nerves, and make the entire body more flexible. Breathing practices increase the body's energy, purify the blood, and nourish the brain. Concentration and meditation techniques clarify the mind and expand awareness. All of these methods contribute to health and mental balance. A daily Yoga practice can include postures, breathing, and meditation, usually accompanied by adherence to a purifying diet. There are certain practices learned by the Yoga student which are performed regularly. Certain postures, for example, are fundamental, and provide overall flexibility and strength. Throughout the course of practice, more advanced postures will be added to the basic routine.

At this point, the similarities and differences between Yoga and Yogatherapy can be examined. Yoga is a system of methods that can be employed by most aspirants. Yogatherapy, however, is a repertoire of specific practices designed to establish health and balance in case of a number of health problems. Almost any health disorder can be relieved to some extent by Yogatherapy. All of the techniques employed in Yogatherapy are from the broader system of Yoga, but they are applied very specifically.

Yoga is an excellent system, geared to the needs of the average practitioner. Yogatherapy is more individually oriented. For particular health problems there are particular Yogic techniques. When these techniques are applied scientifically and in the right order, this is Yogatherapy. Yoga postures, dietary disciplines, and the use of herbs, juices, and food supplements all work together in synergy, restoring balance and health. The specific applications of Yogatherapy are virtually unlimited, with strength and fitness as the results.

The adept sages who developed Yoga many thousands of years ago had a comprehensive working knowledge of anatomy and physiology. This can be verified by looking through some of the traditional Ayurvedic texts. With such a fine understanding, the Yogis were able to create a system of practices which manipulates the form and functions of the body. One posture can improve circulation to the brain, another can stimulate the thyroid, another can loosen the sciatic nerves, and yet another can strengthen the heart. There are Yogic techniques to affect every part of the body, and to relieve every health problem known. There are hundreds of these techniques, many of which have been practiced for centuries.

Yogatherapy as presented here is a systematic approach to the prevention and treatment of many common health problems. Thus the information found here is unique. There are many texts on Yoga, and some are excellent. This book, however, is more than just a general text. This is also a guide for the prevention and treatment of illness. It is of value to those who suffer from ill health, or whose constitution demands preventive therapy. With this book you can adopt a personalized Yoga practice for general health, and can also adopt a personalized Yogatherapy plan to eliminate stress, illness, and tension, and to increase your vitality.

One must approach Yogatherapy with common sense. Yogatherapy is quite effective, and has helped many people. Nonetheless, if you have a serious health problem, it is advisable to seek the advice of a qualified physician who is sympathetic to natural methods of treatment. These people are trained to deal with health and health problems. At the same time, learn to be your own doctor too. Yogatherapy helps to maintain and restore health, while helping a person to develop the sensitivity to perceive the needs of the body. With Yogatherapy you can tune yourself up to enjoy the strength, vigor, sensitivity and vitality which are the marks of vibrant health.

Yogatherapy Can Change Your Life

To some people, health is the absence of disease. Others, however, consider health to be a dynamic, vital state of optimal function. True health is freedom from disease plus energy, joyfulness, and profound vitality. Total health is a condition of living at peak level. Yogatherapy is a means to that kind of health, not merely the absence of disease. It is a powerful system, and if you work with it properly, it will change your life. In this respect, it is a radical departure from other more orthodox health care systems.

Modern medicine tends to view people as fragmented bunches of components and symptoms, and health as the absence of disease. As long as a person doesn't exhibit any clinical pathologies, they are labeled healthy. Even colds, flu, allergies, occasional headaches, pains and low energy are considered par for the course for the average, healthy person. This is a common opinion, because most health care practitioners these days are trained to treat illness and disease, but are not carefully schooled on the factors of radiant health. Thus doctors are often prospecting for disease, rather than considering a way to develop and maintain well-being. Minor ailments are thus accepted as normal. Death is also normal, but premature death is an unnecessary tragedy.

There are small communities in a few isolated parts of the world where disease is unknown, and the people usually live longer than one hundred years. This seems remarkable or fantastic to those of us who live in industrialized societies where virtually everyone suffers some ailment and dies at a much earlier age. The so-called "normal" health disturbances occur only when there is imbalance in the system. Proper exercise, dietary practices, and meditation can create the balance which results in brilliant health. If you are in excellent, radiant health, if energy ripples through you steadily, if you feel and look young, strong, and dynamic, and if you are at ease and free from all tension, then you definitely do not need Yogatherapy. If, on the other hand, you are in less than optimal health, then Yogatherapy is for you. It will help you to reach your peak.

Let me illustrate how powerful Yogatherapy is with a single case history. I was giving a workshop in Boston on health, and several students from one of my Yoga classes were there. Two of the students had brought with them a friend who apparently had a number of health problems. She stayed for the workshop, and afterward we talked at some length. Her name was Janet, and though she had a pretty face, her greatest health problem was obvious. Though she was short, she weighed over two hundred pounds. She felt life a leaf blowing in the wind, as though she had no control over her own life. At that point I told her that she would have to work hard, but that if she would follow my instructions, she would lose weight, become energetic and healthy, and would have tremendous confidence, inner strength, and personal power.

Janet agreed to give it a try, and she started to attend my Yoga classes faithfully, with a daily program at home. At the same time she changed her diet completely according to my specifications. Things changed rapidly for Janet. Over a period of fifteen months, Yogatherapy and Janet's determination radically changed her life. These changes include the following:

- Janet lost over 90 pounds.
- Her energy improved. She used to feel "like slowed down molasses," but she became "super energetic."
- Her eyesight improved, and she wears her glasses less.
- She cut her need for sleep from ten hours nightly to six.
- Menstrual periods were irregular, usually happening only twice a year. With Yogatherapy she became regular, without cramps or discomfort.
- The migraine headaches she had suffered since age two disappeared completely.
- She used to be short of breath, and walking was uncomfortable. In a short period of time, her breathing was normal, she got into the habit of walking a lot, and was able to run comfortably.
- Janet used to wheeze when breathing, and often had to sleep propped up on pillows at night. That cleared up completely.
- Her complexion, once oily with pimples, became clear and healthy looking.
- Her hair was so oily that it had to be washed as much as twice daily. Now it is clean and lustrous.
- Her blood pressure was high, and her pulse used to race. Now both are absolutely normal.
- She has more confidence, feels "centered and more together," and has attained greater peace of mind.

Janet runs a household, has a son and daughter to care for, and operates her own business. With Yogatherapy she has been able to maintain her responsibilities and change her life profoundly at the same time. Her attitude and accomplishments are an inspiration to others, and she is an example of the effectiveness of Yogatherapy.

Now that the ideology and benefits of Yogatherapy have been described, let's turn our attention to some of the essentials of healthy living.

The Mind Body Relationship

Yogis have long understood that the mind and body are thoroughly interwoven, each affecting the other. The mind and body are not in fact separate and distinct, but are interdependant components of the whole person. Throughout the ages the Yogis have emphasized the relationship between the body and mind, and have taught methods for creating a balance. They have long understood that what we think affects the way we feel, and that what we eat, drink and do to our bodies affects the way we think. There can be no separation of function, except for the enlightened adept who has transcended the limitations of the body/mind by assiduous practice of meditation. Even if a condition arises out of what appear to be purely physical circumstances, there will be an accompanying alteration of mood and thought. In addition, thoughts and feelings about a health condition can affect the body's chemistry. Any physical condition will affect the mind in some way. Any state of mind will influence the function of the body.

To understand mind/body interaction more thoroughly, let's examine some clear instances of mind and body affecting each other. When a person drinks an alcoholic beverage, the alcohol acts initially as a stimulant, and then as a sedative hypnotic upon the nervous system. At the same time, mood is often altered. A shy person may become bold and talkative, and the timid may turn aggressive. At a level of intoxication, thinking is impaired, as is motor coordination. There is a clear link between the activity and condition of the body, and changes in mood and behavior.

If a person is given some devastating news, such as the sudden death of a loved one, the person may lose appetite, cry, lose sleep or sleep very heavily, and may experience other physical phenomena such as diarrhea and sweating. In this instance, information provided to the mind triggers a drastic alteration of physical function.

When a runner trains to run long distances, a phenomenon known as "runner's high" may develop. After running for several miles, a person may start to feel high, or euphoric, and may experience a sense of tremendous mental well-being. This is due to the fact that many long distance runners produce large quantities of endorphins in the brain. Endorphins are morphine-like substances, and they produce the elated state that many runners experience.

Mental anxiety, a common symptom of today's overpressured people, is frequently relieved by administration of diazepam, a prescription drug so effective (but addictive) that it earned the name "mother's little helper." Here a pill taken by the body alters (an apparently) mental condition.

Individuals trained in the techniques of biofeedback can alter their own brain-wave activity, and can create changes in the incipient sweating of their pores. They can also modify the temperature of their hands.

Pheromones, subtle chemicals which are manufactured by the body, act as powerful sexual attractants. Though pheromones are odorless, they are picked up by subtle receptors in the human olfactory (sense of smell) mechanism. Pheromones provoke sexual attraction, and all of the accompanying mental states associated with that attraction.

A chemical called LHRH (luteinizing-hormone releasing hormone) is manufactured in the body, and is a powerful sexual stimulant. Some people secrete more LHRH than most others do. These individuals fall in love very quickly and intensely, over and over again. Their short, dramatic relationships are often punctuated by intensely passionate sexual activity. When these people are given a drug which inhibits LHRH, their behavior changes considerably, and they no longer experience the same intense, frenzied romantic/sexual urges.

Certain food additives have been known to cause chemically induced psychosis.

Artificial colors, flavors, and preservatives can produce schizophrenia in some individuals, while having seemingly no effect upon others.

Nutritionally, there are many known body/mind interactions. Blood sugar is the amount of glucose in the bloodstream. This is the fuel used by the body. The B-complex vitamins and the mineral zinc are involved in the regulation of blood sugar. An imbalance in these nutrients can result in an imbalance of blood sugar. This frequently results in behavioral changes such as irritability, depression, lack of clarity, and in some cases, schizophrenia. These mental states have been successfully treated in many cases by providing adequate amounts of nutrients to the body.

Phosphatidylcholine, a concentrate of lecithin, has been shown to enhance the production of a brain chemical called *acetylcholine*. Acetylcholine is important to memory function. There are many reports of improved memory function due to consumption of lecithin and its concentrate, phosphatidylcholine.

Is there a separation between the body and mind, or are they components of one organic whole? The Yogis say that there is no separation. The body and mind are interwoven, interfunctional, and interdependant. The conditioning of the body will have a positive influence not only upon physical fitness, but upon mood and mental fitness as well. Likewise, the training of the mind will not only sharpen mental acuity, but will also benefit the body.

Yogis with excellent self-control can remain in particular postures for extended periods of time. A recent case in point is that of Herakhan Baba, who in 1970 seated himself in a meditation position, and did not move for 45 days. During that time he did not eat, sleep, speak, or go to the bathroom. Granted, this is an extraordinary example of control, but it effectively illustrates the point. Mahatma Gandhi had sufficient control over his body and mind that he sat awake and chatted with doctors while his appendix was removed without the use of any anesthesia or pain killers. Many Yogis and adepts have demonstrated the ability to change the patterns of brainwaves, alter pulse rate and body temperature, eliminate pain, and even walk on fire. These people insist that it is mental training that enables them to perform such feats.

The Yogatherapy approach to health considers the mind/body as one integrated whole. In working with Yogatherapy, one works with the mind and body together. For example, to improve digestion, postures will be used to affect the stomach, liver, and intestines. At the same time, breathing techniques can refresh the mind and reduce stress. Meditation can clear the mind, calm the nervous system, and benefit the digestive process. Dietary changes affect brain/body chemistry, and contribute to a greater mental and physical balance. To truly heal, Yogatherapy approaches the body and mind as inseparable.

A consideration of the mind/body relationship inevitably leads to an examination of so-called "superhuman" abilities of the body and mind, such as the extraordinary physical and mental control described previously. While the ability to control bodily function, eliminate pain, or change the activity of the brain is surely impressive, such talents are neither supernatural nor unattainable. We possess remarkable minds, yet we use just a fraction of our mind power in daily living. In the section on

Meditation, there are techniques for harnessing greater mind power. You need not shave your head, wear a turban, or turn yourself into a living scarecrow through austerities to develop a strong meditation practice. You must simply practice daily, persistently. If you want to become a good runner, you must train regularly. If you want to develop your mind/body potential, then the regular practice of Yoga and meditation can enable you to attain that goal.

Yogatherapy offers an opportunity to improve your health while expanding your horizons. Almost everyone wants more energy, strength, mental clarity, and personal satisfaction. Yogatherapy offers a way to approach the mind/body to derive the maximum benefit for your efforts. Just as there is no end to human potential, there is no end to self-fulfillment. Yogatherapy is a means toward ever-greater fulfillment of the mind/body.

Yoga Philosophy

Yoga means Union, an integration of oneself, and at-oneness with Nature, all of creation, and with the Absolute. The very word Yoga defines the goal of life as understood by the great Yogic sages of India. The practice of the various systems of Yoga is the means by which the realization of Union can be attained. This is an important point; the goal is not to achieve Union. Union, or oneness with the creation and the Creator, is our prior, fundamental condition. The aim of Yoga is to bring to fruition the realization of that Union. We are already at one with the Universe; we just don't know it.

The path of Yoga is predicated on the understanding that all things in the Universe are connected and interrelated. This same assumption is now part and parcel of the science of physics. From the Yogic point of view, the Universe is not a fragmented conglomeration in which man is separate from nature and the Divine. Instead, the Universe is seen as a multidimensional and integrated expression of the Creator. The Absolute, or the Creator, is the essence and origin of all things. According to the Yogis, the Creator and the creation are one, indivisible. There are not two; there is only One.

At this point it is necessary to interject that Yoga is definitely not a religion. Though culturally linked to both Hinduism and Buddhism, Yoga stands on its own, and is free from all separatist and dualistic attitudes of religion. People of all religions (or of no religion) can engage in Yoga practice. For though the meditative practices of Yoga are profound and revelatory in nature, they are not limited by the notions of any systems of beliefs. Yoga is based on the direct perception of all the Truths it espouses, and does not rely upon ritual and dogma to remain vital and timely. Naturally, many individuals, groups, sects, and cults have added their own beliefs, rituals, ceremonies, and dogma to the Way of Yoga. But in its purest form, Yoga is beyond all such trappings.

Conventional notions of God conjure images of a male or female figure, estranged and separate from all else, sitting in heaven while keeping a watchful eye on things down below. This separatist view differentiates between the Creator and creation. This is unacceptable to the Yogic philosophy, which is founded upon Union. The Creator is the original, unmanifest, primordial essence of the Universe, from which all creation emerges, and into which it is ultimately dissolved.

It follows, then, that we and the Creator are one. It is not the case that anyone is Divine to the exclusion of others, but that Divinity is our essential nature. This can be perceived only by direct experience. No amount of cleverness, reading, or speculation can make this understanding apparent to us. Realization comes with diligent practice of Yoga. The Goal and the Path are one and the same.

When we consider the Absolute, we are dealing with that which is limitless, eternal, without beginning or end, omniscient, omnipresent, and thoroughly beyond human comprehension. Our Divinity is infinite, and that understanding cannot be held by the finite mind, which is limited by habitual thoughts, feelings, and conceptions. To know the infinite is to know the unknowable. To do that requires that we undergo a tremendous transformation. Such revolutionary change is possible by treading the Yogic path, by meditating and directing oneself toward ultimate understanding. Yoga, which is Union with the Absolute, is attained through Yoga, the path of Union. The goal and the path are one, inseparable.

According to the Yogic philosophy, we are all here to tread the path of knowledge and realization. The purpose of life is to expand our consciousness in order to eventually realize and manifest our natural Divinity. This evolutionary scheme is set in the scenery of life as we know it, a life whose conditions and circumstances are present to fuel the fire of growth. According to the Yogis, all of our life experiences are useful to facilitate our gradual awakening to Cosmic Consciousness and the thorough realization of our Divinity. Every situation and circumstance in life in some manner helps us along the Path. We have the capacity to be self-aware, and to apply our conscious gifts to the attainment of self-mastery, which leads to the transcendent awareness which leads to the realization of Divinity. This great awakening, this transcendent understanding, is illumination, or Enlightenment. Enlightenment is the true experience of Yoga, or Union.

To understand the undertaking of being consciously "on the Path," we must examine some further aspects of Yogic Philosophy. One essential aspect of this is reincarnation. Reincarnation is the process by which an individual soul incarnates, or is embodied, in successive lives, and as distinctly different beings. According to this understanding, we are at our very essence Souls, fundamentally spiritually beings. We incarnate many thousands of times, in a variety of forms.

There is currently a great deal of misunderstanding and sensationalism about reincarnation. We can thank the lesser writers of occult fantasy for that. In addition, many people hotly dispute the actuality of such a scheme. How can one truly know the existence and nature of reincarnation? The only way to know, is to experience. We are fortunate to live at a time when techniques are available by which one can directly experience past incarnations. This experience opens up tremendous new vistas of awareness, because it enables one to see oneself as an everlasting soul with many different identities, each as real as the one we are experiencing right now. It is a revolutionary insight into existence, and having had the experience, one can never be the same.

Each incarnation, each appearance, each lifetime, affords an opportunity to learn different lessons in life, to have particular experiences, and to help us each to begin to awaken in our own peculiar way. An identity and a life is much like a suit of clothing, worn for a particular occasion, and then discarded. The life is over, the personality dissolves, yet the soul remains. One can say that even more fundamental than the understanding of reincarnation is the realization of immortality. As part of the Creator, a person is spirit everlasting. Life is the vehicle used to learn the secrets of existence, and to tread the Path.

According to the great Yogic sages, Patanjali, Siva, Buddha, and others, the whole Universe is evolving. All that is manifest is growing toward full awareness of Divinity. This process takes aeons and aeons to be completed. Buddha was asked by one of his disciples how long it had taken for humanity to evolve to the point at which it had arrived thus far. Buddha's answer was this: Imagine that there is a mountain made of stone, and that mountain is a mile high and ten miles wide. Once every hundred years an eagle flies over the mountain, making just one pass. In the beak of the eagle is a fine silk scarf. As the eagle passes over the mountain, the scarf brushes lightly against the peak. We have been evolving for as long as it would take to wear the mountain down to nothing with the scarf.

The illustration is dramatic, and it serves the purpose of conveying that we have been around for a long, long time. And it is a great and auspicious occasion when at last we become self-aware enough to enquire into the meaning and purpose of life. We may pass through several lifetimes of questioning and speculation, but the real turning point comes when we turn to some means by which we can directly apprehend the truth. Yoga is such a means, a Path of Union and Enlightenment.

It must be understood, however, that the classical Yogic disciplines are not the only means for such realization. Many cultures have developed paths of knowledge. There is no monopoly on truth and awareness; wherever there are people, there will be some way to expand, evolve, and fulfill oneself. All of these paths have different forms and practices, but the eventual realization is the same.

A question which naturally arises is at what point does a person become aware enough to consciously embark upon the Path, and how can you account for the tremendous variations in human awareness? Why do some people become more aware than others? The answer lies in another cornerstone of the Yogic philosophy, the doctrine of *Karma*.

Karma is the law of cause and effect. The basic premise of *karma* is the principle that for every action there is an equal and opposite reaction. *Karma* is the principle that whatever we are and do evokes an exactly appropriate response from the rest of the Universe. We may be confused, perplexed, or unaware of why certain things happen, but they do so in order to maintain a balance of forces as we move through life. *Karma* is the force that Jesus described, when he said "As you sow, so shall you reap."

The Judeo-Christian tradition envisions a scheme of Divine retribution, a system of checks and balances managed by an anthropomorphic God. The notion that there is a heavenly being who dutifully doles out punishment or rewards according to our conduct is both romantic and egocentric. *Karma* is a universal force, affecting each of us individually as it affects all beings collectively. It is a natural Cosmic law of physics, and is identical to the principles of Sir Isaac Newton.

What does *karma* mean to us? How does it affect us, and what has it to do with our evolution toward Enlightenment? According to Yoga philosophy, the tendency toward the awakening of the self is the primary operating force within us. *Karma*, on the other hand, is the force which helps us along the way and makes us pay as we go. All our actions, thoughts, words and feelings have an effect upon us and the environment. Everything that is a part of us creates an effect in some way. This effect, however strong or subtle, sets in motion forces which respond to that effect in an appropriate way. Our life circumstances reflect both the forces that we have generated, and what we need to further evolve. We are not isolated from each other or from the world. Everything which occurs anywhere affects all of us, however subtly. This conclusion is part of the new physics; everything is connected to everything else. Humanity as a whole reaps the collective pains and rewards of its own actions. World trends or movements are a mass *karmic* effect. Adolf Hitler, for example, could find and mobilize the destructive and maniacal forces which are part of the dark side of humanity. On the other hand, a force like Gandhi can mobilize a great good within millions of people, and can initiate a movement toward peace and humanitarian consciousness that will last long after he has passed away. Everybody leaves their mark. A rare few change the world in a grand manner.

Individually *karma* enables us to grow and learn, propelling us onward, while demanding that we achieve resolution with every circumstance of which we are a part. A person who is kind, loving and generous will at some point be the object of those same forces, whereas a person who is hateful, greedy and cruel will ultimately be forced to deal with the same. In some way, each of us reaps what we have sown.

This is where an understanding of reincarnation comes into play. It is immediately apparent that many people do not seem to reap what they have sown. More than one generous servant of humanity has suffered or died cruelly, or has been denied recognition or reward for a life of selfless service. Many such people have endured great pain to perform their work. On the other hand, there are plenty of fat cats who have taken horrible advantage of others, and in doing so have reaped wealth, comfort, and privilege, with no apparent pains or obstacles. Things do not always happen in one lifetime. *Karma* is a complex system of checks and balances which operates over a generous period of time. We carry accumulated *karma* from life to life, working out old *karma* as we create it anew. Thus the unsung servant of humanity may be exalted in the next lifetime. Or perhaps that person served and suffered due to a previous lifetime spree of excess and vainglory. The fat cat of today may be the destitute pauper of tomorrow.

Karma, being an impersonal Cosmic force, is the ultimate justice. We are guaranteed to receive whatever we are due, no more, no less. At the same time, our natural evolutionary tendency pushes us on to greater awareness as we work with and through our *karma*. It is *karma* that accounts for the tremendous differences in human awareness and development on the evolutionary scale. We assist or impede our evolution by the way that we live and think. What we do with our lives determines how we will grow. It is a matter of choice, set within the context of circumstances that are a response to past *karmic* accumulations.

Ignorance clouds the mind and obscures clear vision, keeping us unaware of the great joy and ecstasy of Enlightenment. But at some point there is enough realization to investigate the purpose of life. Then *karma* becomes a tool to guide us to the information or person that gives us our first glimpse of the Path. From that point on, the process of evolutionary growth is accelerated and becomes more demanding. With greater awareness comes increased responsibility for our thoughts, feelings, and conduct. Then growth becomes a conscious process, not a haphazard string of events which happen to us. We face ourselves with more clarity, every day assuming more responsibility for who we are and what we do.

The road to Mastery as described in the Yogic philosophy is both arduous and exciting. It is arduous because the task is overwhelming. Every possible distraction, diversion, and obstacle stands in the way of our conscious growth. The entire world with its fascinating and intriguing phenomena is *Maya*. *Maya* is the ancient Sanskrit word for the Great Dance of Illusion. The Yogic Path is a fierce and powerful means for cutting through that illusion, and breaking through to full self-realization. The excitement of this lies in the revelation that we are all Creators. We create the circumstances and conditions of our lives. With clarity, focused intent, and determination, we can create whatever we want. This creative power is limited only by our perceptual boundaries. The more expanded our awareness becomes, the more powerfully we can consciously manifest our own reality.

Yoga philosophy is vast and complex, while it is underscored by a few basic principles. We have examined some of these key elements enough to develop a feeling for the conceptual framework of Yoga practice. For although this is primarily a book on health, an examination of Yoga philosophy is very useful. It can only enhance the value of our endeavors.

Life and Energy

Life is energy. Life is an ongoing expression of various forces which are constantly interacting. There is nothing static about life; it is a continuous interplay of energy from many sources. Life is always growing, changing, reforming, creating, regenerating, and moving on.

The single, original source of all life is the one, Absolute, Eternal Creator of the Universe. But as the Universe has sprung forth into countless forms, there have come to be many ways by which energy is channeled and directed. Thus there have come to be many sources of energy which support life. Energy can be electrical, atomic, chemical, thermal, physical, or of some other nature, depending upon the form it assumes. There are endless ways by which energy is generated, channeled, and released.

We humans are very complex, and we rely on several different means by which we receive energy to support life in an optimal manner. The various components of our being require different energies to function well. These energies all work together in synergy, and when they are balanced correctly, there is excellent health and well-being. Some of the primary energies that we need are as follow:

SPIRIT: The highest aspect of a human being is the spirit, which is the most refined and direct link to the pure, unmanifest creative energy of the Universe. It is the human spirit which is the bridge between mortality and immortality, and between the finite and the infinite. Spirit is the first and most fundamental energy for life.

MIND: We are intelligent beings. Our sophisticated intelligence enables us to think, to make choices, and to live life strategically. Mental energy directly feeds and nourishes the mind, the seat of human intelligence. It is the great power of mind which gives us a keen edge in life. Without mental energy we would have no creative intelligence, and would live purely at a survival level.

EMOTION: One of the most powerful human energies is emotion. Emotion is that power by which we intensify, magnify, and feel the experiences of life. The feeling of emotion is a sense which touches us in our innermost core. Emotional feeling gives people a sense of being involved and associated with life, rather than being casual outside observers. Emotion is a unique function of the mind, and is a powerful enriching element in relationships between people.

VITALITY: There is energy which is neither mental, emotional, nor purely physical. This energy is known as vitality. Each person has a complex energy system, often referred to as the vitality body, or the etheric body. This aspect of the human mind/body is the fundamental energetic substructure upon which the dense physical body is built. The vitality body is a bright, egg-shaped, luminous body of fine energy channels, very similar in appearance to the physical nervous system. These energy channels, called *nadis*, are the pathways through which vital energy flows. Such energy may come from the breath, from the sun, from meditation practice, or other sources. Where these energy channels meet, there are intense vortices of energy. These vortices are called *chakras*, which are described in more detail later on.

PHYSICAL: This energy is the most dense form of life sustenance. Most physical energy is received via the food we eat, and through what we drink. The physical body relies upon the chemical and physical constituents of these substances for life energy. The physical body is directly affected by whatever occurs in the Spirit, Mind, Emotions, or Vitality Body. In turn, the physical body can affect the other aspects of our total constitution.

The Aura

Surrounding every human being is a field of life energy known as the *aura*. The *aura* is the subject of much investigation, and it has been photographed, measured, examined, and studied. The Yogis have long known that the *aura* is a statement—in visible and colorful life energy—of who and what we are, what we feel, and how we think. The *aura* is like an energy fingerprint, unique to each individual. Many people easily and readily see *auras*, although most people do not.

The *aura* is a human rainbow body. It is colorful, and each color has a different meaning, indicating particular factors about a person. The size, shape, brilliance, and colors of the *aura* are all determined by who we are, and by how we feel. A very vital, positive, dynamic person will have a correspondingly brilliant, gleaming, large *aura*. On the other hand, a miserable, energy-less, sickly person will have a dull, thin, unappealing *aura*. Often it is the *aura* which makes us feel a person's presence, though not a word may be said.

The *aura* is also a shield. It is a semi-permeable membrane, through which certain types of energy may pass. A brilliant, strong *aura* will let in only the most positive and health giving energies, while deflecting less healthful forces. A weak, thin *aura*, however, will let in all manner of psychic garbage. Yogatherapy, in both its physical and meditative aspects, helps to build a strong, gleaming, radiant *aura*. This is a reflection of dynamic health, and makes one accessible to only the finest of life supporting forces.

Perfect Health Is a Perfect Balance of Energy: All the different factors and energies previously described must function together in a balanced and harmonious fashion if health is to be maintained. If there is either excess or a lack of any particular energy, or if living habits do not accommodate true needs, then there will be imbalance. Health is a total state. It is the result of an interplay of many factors.

Yogatherapy emphasizes the need for balance. We must not neglect our bodies for our minds, nor must we neglect our minds for our bodies, as health is an ongoing state of staying in balance. People must learn to be aware of their needs, and must tend to those needs in an intelligent manner. True intelligence is a continuous creative process. It is not just the accumulation of information. Any small computer, even a pocket calculator, can store and retrieve information. What makes people different is creativity. We can use information in millions of ways. We can tune in to the source of all life, energy, and intelligence. With such attunement, health is entirely attainable, and health can be common fare.

Illness, or Dis-ease Is an Imbalance of Energy: If we are out of balance, if we are not living in harmony with the laws of Nature and with our own needs, then illness results. Whether by eating to excess, living with regular anger, or denying ourselves total nourishment of the mind/body, we generate sickness. There are no magic cures, no instant pills, potions, or panaceas. The way of health is a way of life, and treatments and cures are proportionate to the severity of whatever disease state may exist. The more aware one can be, the more resources there are to work with to remain healthy and vibrant. Most people accept decay, degeneration, and sickness as unavoidable components of life. But this is only because we have been educated in an imbalanced manner. We have been taught to accept disease and imbalance as part of life, and so we do. What would happen if we didn't? Don't allow yourself to be hypnotized by that way of thinking. Your determined refusal to accept the philosophy of degeneration will enable you to open up new worlds of possibility for yourself. Then health is a possibility.

Imbalances can be corrected by applying understanding and the resources available to us. The first step toward health is to accept health and balance as a realistic and desirable possibility. From that point of departure, Yogatherapy can provide you with practical tools to make health and vibrance real for you.

The Chakras

As stated before, there are vortices of energy in the body known as *chakras*. While there are many points of concentrated energy within the entire mind/body system, there are seven chakras in particular which are considered to be the major centers of energy within each human being. Through the chakras, all types of life energy flow. Through each single chakra, energy is directed to corresponding organs, glands, and nerves. In addition, each chakra is associated with particular aspects of human consciousness. The First Chakra, for example, which is located at the root of the spinal column, is associated with survival, while the Fifth Chakra, located in the throat, is associated with higher creativity. All of the aspects of human function and human consciousness are associated with the chakras.

The seven major vortices of energy function together as one complex energy system. In the entire mind/body system, everything works together with everything else. Nothing is separate and distinct from all else. Human beings are amazing examples of the cooperation of various forces. The chakras are involved with every possible aspect of human function. And the chakras, like organs and glands, can be weak or strong, and can work well or function poorly. The optimal condition is for these vortices to be at peak level of function, in a perfect balance with one another. This happens when one leads a balanced life. A "balanced life" is different for everyone, as we are all unique. It is our task in life to figure out exactly what that balance is, and to live by that, allowing for the continuous changes which occur.

A detailed exposition of the chakras is not necessary for the purposes of Yogatherapy, but some facts are useful. Since the chakras are associated with specific organs, glands, nerves, and aspects of human consciousness, they are very much associated with health. Everything you do has an effect upon the condition of the chakras. This in turn has an effect upon energy flow, which in turn influences mind/

body function. The following is a description of the consciousness associated with each of the seven major energy vortices. That is followed by a chart describing anatomical and functional correlations.

The First Chakra: This energy center is associated with the most basic aspects of human energy and survival. The energy that flows through the First Chakra is dense, vital, and powerful. Survival is an urge which underlies almost all human behavior. For in order to do anything else, we must survive. Just as the First Chakra is at the root of the spine, so is the conscious influence of the First Chakra at the root of all human behavior.

The Second Chakra: Creativity occurs in many ways, at many levels. The most fundamental creativity is the act of procreation through sexual activity. The Second Chakra is the center of sexual energy, of basic creativity and regeneration. Sexual energy, because it is a creative force, can be expressed in millions of ways. This is why sexuality influences thought, feelings, behavior, art, music, fashion, even architecture and automobile manufacturing! Sexual orgasm is both a basic experience of profound biological satisfaction, and at the same time a transcendent experience. The Second Chakra is a highly active energy center whose energy permeates virtually everything else that we are and do. It is basic creativity, also associated with survival of the species, while at the same time being connected to ecstatic feelings of the highest order.

The Third Chakra: This is the strongest center of the individual self, and of the Will. Beyond basic survival and continuation of the species, there is individuation of consciousness, in which we experience ourselves as unique beings. The Third Chakra is the focal area of that expression, the center from which we experience our own personal power. Will, or the power of personal determination, originates from this energy vortex. Through the Third Chakra flows the energy of self assertion, personal direction, and individual strength. It is with this energy that we have the force to move and grow and meet challenges in the world. The Third Chakra can be enormously powerful, and is associated with what is frequently referred to as *charisma*.

The Fourth Chakra: Known as the center of Love and compassion, the fourth vortex of energy offers a radical departure in consciousness from the first three, as it is the first center of attention to other than oneself. The energy that flows through this center is directed, not just toward personal survival, but beyond, to the consideration of other beings. Thus the Fourth Chakra is truly a center of expanded awareness, of connection with the rest of the world. This center is also the midpoint between the lower three centers and the higher three, and is the conscious point of departure from one to another. It is through the awareness of the Fourth Chakra that we gain access to our highest awareness and creativity.

The Fifth Chakra: The energy for the higher functions of creativity, artistic expression, and speech flow through this center. The force of the Fifth Chakra is most noticeable in the activity of speech. One can speak with tremendous force and influence when this center is well developed. Speech may well be the single most influential human behavior known. All creative activity, from painting to writing to playing music, involves a process by which we express something from within. When creative energies of the Fifth Chakra are strong, such expression can be dramatic, powerful, and deeply moving. The force from this center can literally be spellbinding.

The Sixth Chakra: Also known as the Third Eye, or Wisdom Eye, this energy vortex is the location of higher intelligence and supranormal vision. In the truest and most literal sense, the Third Eye is the center of insight, an inner vision accompanied by wisdom and deep understanding of the subtle forces at play in any situation. When the Third Eye is "open," one can see the past, present, and future clearly, in a continuum. Individuals with this extraordinary vision are the few true clairvoyants and sages who have lived among humanity throughout history. The higher intelligence associated with the Sixth Chakra is one accompanied by great sensitivity to a balance of all energies, at all times. Such vision enables a person to live and behave in a manner which promotes the most positive possible outcomes in all situations.

The Seventh Chakra: Cosmic consciousness is a state of absolute awareness of and integration with the primary, creative force of the Universe. This unconditional state of total freedom, wisdom, energy, insight, and joy, is the natural human condition upon the full and total awakening of the Seventh Chakra. Such full awakening is usually the product of many successive lifetimes of purification, inner refinement, and spiritual work. However, that does not mean that cosmic consciousness is unavailable to one who has not undergone such training. The Universe is vast and mysterious, and there is more to it than fits into any one philosophy, school, or body of knowledge. The ways to supreme ecstasy are many. Knowing how to love and being joyful seem to be the two most fundamental keys to growing into an unlimited Cosmic state. So don't worry yourself with the complications of dogma and exotic philosophies. Just be happy, and learn to Love.

Chakra Chart

1st Chakra
Location: Base of spine, at perineum, between anus and genitals.
Name: *Muladhara*
Associated organs: Large intestine, rectum
Associated glands: Adrenal glands

Primary nerves: Sacral plexus
Primary functions: Survival, power, vital life energy, elimination.

2nd Chakra
Location: At spine, close to genitals.
Name: *Svadhisthana*
Associated organs: Large intestine, bladder, kidneys, genitals.
Associated glands: All glands associated with sex organs.
Primary nerves: (male) prostatic plexus, (female) utero-vaginal plexus.
Primary functions: Survival, procreation, vital life energy, sexual function.

3rd Chakra
Location: At spine, across from solar plexus.
Name: *Manipura*
Associated organs: Liver, spleen, stomach, small intestine.
Associated glands: Pancreas
Primary nerves: Solar plexus
Primary functions: Will, personal power, digestion, assimilation of nutrients

4th Chakra
Location: At spine, across from sternum.
Name: *Anahata*
Associated organs: Heart, lungs.
Associated glands: Thymus gland
Primary nerves: Cardiac plexus
Primary functions: Love, compassion, immunity, heart, lung, and bronchial functions.

5th Chakra
Location: At spine, at throat.
Name: *Visuddha*
Associated organs: Vocal cords
Associated glands: Thyroid gland
Primary nerves: Pharyngeal plexus
Primary functions: Higher creativity, speech.

6th Chakra
Location: Center of head
Name: *Ajna*
Associated organs: Brain
Associated glands: Pituitary gland
Primary nerves: Cavernous plexus
Primary functions: Higher intelligence, clairvoyance, insight, refined hearing.

7th Chakra
Location: Center of head
Name: *Sahasrara*
Associated organs: Brain
Associated glands: Pineal gland
Primary nerves: Cavernous plexus
Primary functions: Cosmic consciousness

Including Yogatherapy in Your Daily Plan

To include Yogatherapy in your daily schedule may take a little rearranging of your daily plan, but it is necessary to do so with anything that requires regular involvement. Depending on the Yogatherapy program you are on, there will be exercise and dietary plans to follow daily, as well as meditation.

There are three times in the day which seem to be optimal for Yogatherapy practice. The best time is in the morning, upon rising, because practice at that time will set the tone for the rest of the day. If you have trouble getting started in the morning, this will take some getting used to. But once you have gotten into such a schedule, you will find that you have more energy than you would have gotten from sleeping later. A hot and cold shower will also help, and then your Yoga program will give you extra energy, and a fresh, ready-to-go feeling.

Late afternoon seems to be another good time. Perhaps it is not possible for you to fit your program in first thing in the day. The late afternoon is a good alternate time, as you can refresh yourself at that time, and have more energy for the rest of the day and evening.

The third time seems to be late in the evening. Some people find this the best time to practice. This is also a peaceful time, and you will find that sleep will be deep and satisfying.

Whatever your game plan is, make sure that you allow yourself enough time to do your Yogatherapy program fully and correctly. Self health care is a process that involves a commitment to personal well-being and growth. You may even find that you will have to sacrifice some other activity to accommodate your pursuit of Yogatherapy. That is just part of making changes. Very few things provide comparable energy, health, and a feeling of well-being.

Yogatherapy is something which will add new dimensions to the rest of your day, and to the rest of your life. Include it faithfully in your way of life, and you will be well rewarded.

Advice on the Practice
of Yogatherapy Exercises and Postures

- Be sure that you are clean when you practice. Preferably, take a shower before hand. Otherwise, at least wash your hands, face and feet prior to practice.
- Practice when you have time—do not hurry.
- Always practice on an empty stomach, not sooner than three hours after having eaten.
- Practice in a place that is neither too hot nor too cold.
- Never practice on a hard surface. Use a mat, rug, blanket, or pad.
- If possible, set aside a place just for Yogatherapy practice. Keep it bright, clean, and peaceful.
- Practice in a well ventilated area.
- If possible, practice where there are few distractions around you.
- Whenever you can, practice outside where it is clean and fresh. A secluded, grassy spot is ideal.
- Wear loose, non-restrictive clothing. This should be light weight, cotton clothing.
- The less clothing the better. Practicing in minimal clothing gives you more freedom to move.

When Yogatherapy Is Not Recommended

If a person is critically ill, particularly when the condition is life-threatening, then Yogatherapy is not recommended. In such cases, one should be in the care of a competent physician. At this point in time, there are increasingly many doctors who are sympathetic to a holistic approach to health. If you can find such a person, then that is ideal. Even if you can't, however, a life-threatening illness necessitates the care of a qualified medical doctor.

Yogatherapy is a highly effective health care system, but like anything, it has its limits. Just as a person with a serious gunshot wound would not seek chiropractic care for that problem, so too an individual in serious crisis should not choose that time to begin self health care without expert guidance. Your doctor may approve of some involvement with the therapies described here, or may prefer that you wait until you are somewhat recovered. In any case, be judicious with your involvement. A little bit of emergency medical care during a crisis will enable you to pursue alternatives on your own later.

Learning to Breathe

Breath is life. With every breath, you draw pure, life energy into yourself. This energy, known as *prana*, circulates through the entire human bioenergetic system, promoting life and health.

Proper breathing is an essential component of Yogatherapy. One must learn to breathe correctly, deeply, and easily, to gain maximum benefit from the breath, and to promote dynamic health. Many people actually have to relearn how to breathe correctly, because improper breathing habits are common. It is important to correct this, and to learn to breathe in a natural manner. Breath is very nourishing, and when you breathe correctly, you can feel the vitality and power of each breath you take.

For the purposes of the materials presented in this book, we will work with only two methods of breathing. There are dozens of breathing techniques in Yoga, all of which serve different functions. But we will limit ourselves to the two most essential breaths of all. One is the normal breath, and the other is the long, deep breath. Both of these breaths are used in the Yogatherapy techniques described later on.

The Normal Breath: Sit in a comfortable position, either cross-legged or in a straight chair. Let your spine be erect, so that you are sitting tall and straight. The shoulders and chest are relaxed. Place one hand on your abdomen. Take a light breath through the nose, and as you do, let the abdomen extend outward. The chest should not move much at all. It is like filling a balloon. As you inhale, the abdomen expands. As you exhale, it collapses. This is very important. Go over this again and again. Breath is one of the keys to Yogatherapy, and it must be employed correctly. For about two minutes, practice easy, gentle breathing, expanding the abdominal area as you inhale, and letting it collapse as you exhale. This is the relaxed breath that you should maintain during the day.

Note: It is important to inhale through the nose, as inhaling through the mouth bypasses energy regulating mechanisms in the body, and can lead to imbalances which may generate physical and emotional problems. Be sure always to inhale through the nose. Exhalation may be either through the mouth or nose.

The Long Deep Breath: This is similar to the normal breath, except that it is deeper. This time, put one hand on your abdomen, and one in the middle of your chest. This is for practice only. As you take a breath, fill your abdomen as before in the normal breath. After this is filled, continue to inhale until your lungs are full. Your chest will rise and expand as you do so. Then gently exhale and let the breath out. It is important that you work with this breath until you do it correctly, easily. This breath is very much like filling a glass of water. You pour water in from the top, but the glass fills from the bottom up. It is the same with the breath. You breathe from the top of your body, but you fill up from your lower abdomen, and then your chest. You fill with breath from the bottom up. Practice this for a few minutes every day, until you have perfected the breath. Breath is life—use it to your advantage.

Yoga Postures and Exercises

Soorya Namaskar—Salute to the Sun

Salute to the Sun is one of the fundamental practices of Hatha Yoga, and is considered to be extremely beneficial. Having worked with this for several years, I can only heartily agree. Salute to the Sun is a complete Yoga practice in itself. If you do nothing else but add this to your daily plan, you will feel stronger, healthier, and more alive. This is because Salute to the Sun stretches you out front to back, and energizes you all over. As with most of what we do in Yogatherapy, the motions in this are integrated with the breath. Thus, as you move, you stretch out, tone up, and charge yourself with prana from the breath.

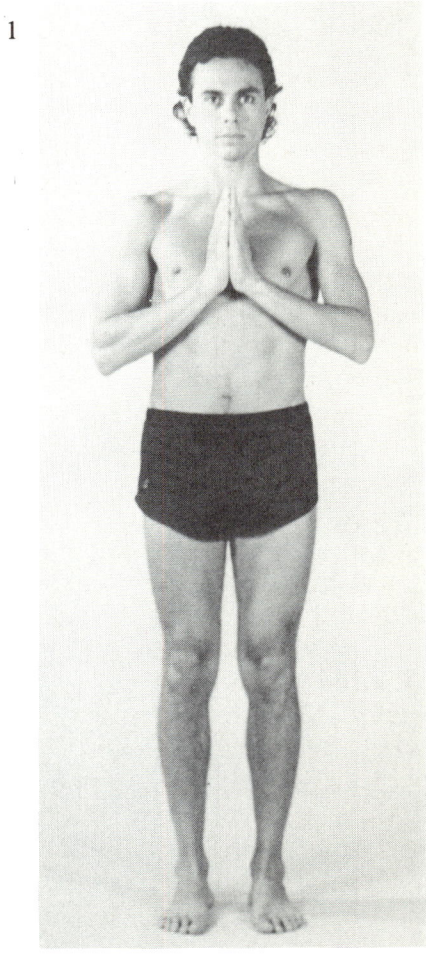

1

There is only one precaution which should be observed here. If you are new to Yoga, or are not used to a lot of backward bending, then do not bend back too far in the standing position. Later on as your back becomes stronger and you are more flexible, you will be able to stretch back as far as you like with no difficulty.

Start out doing this three to five times a day, as the first part of your daily Yogatherapy practice. Gradually build up until you do Salute to the Sun eight or ten times in a row. It is a most remarkable practice, and will yield the finest results.

Directions:
1. Stand straight with the palms together at the chest. Feet are two or three inches apart.
2. Inhale, stretching up and back. Let

head stretch back.
3. Exhale forward and down, bringing hands beside feet.
4. Inhale, stretching your left leg back, with your head up.
5. Exhale, stretching right leg back, bring body into a triangle. Head is down, chin tucked in.
6. Inhale forward and down, with chin, chest, knees and toes touching the ground. Hips are off the ground, with the buttocks up.
7. Hold the breath, as you drop the hips to the ground, push the arms straight, and stretch back into Cobra pose.

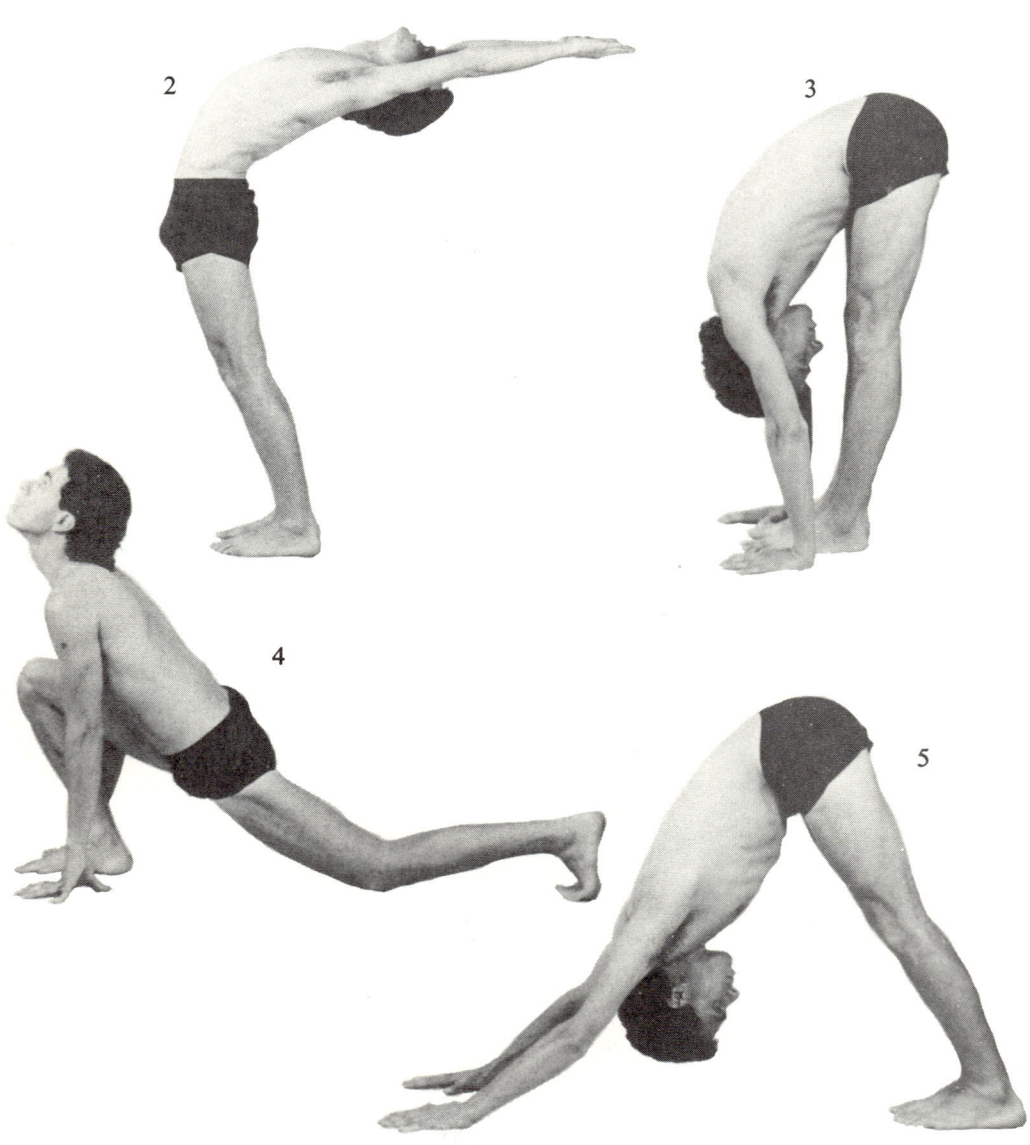

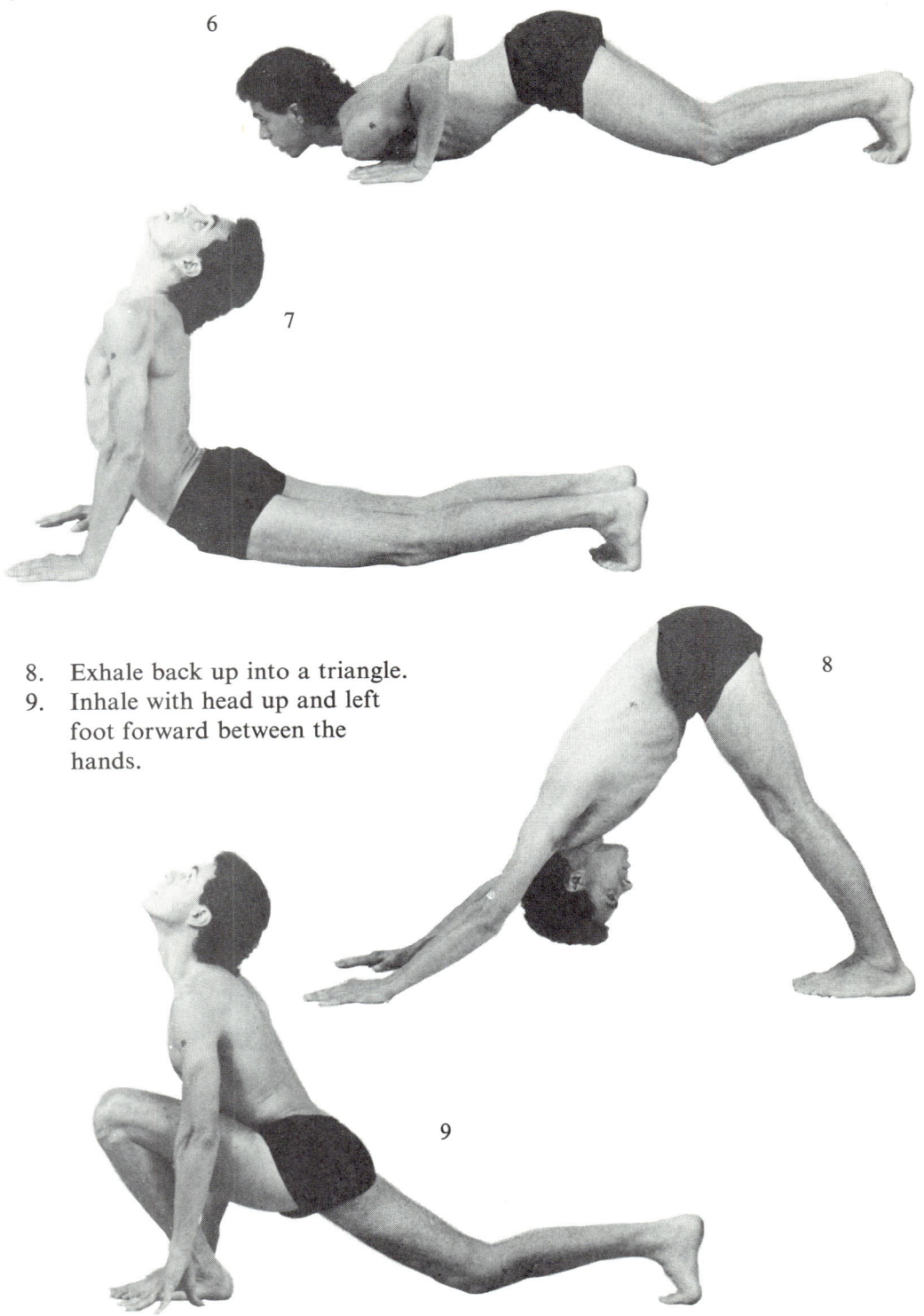

8. Exhale back up into a triangle.
9. Inhale with head up and left foot forward between the hands.

42/Yoga and Yogatherapy

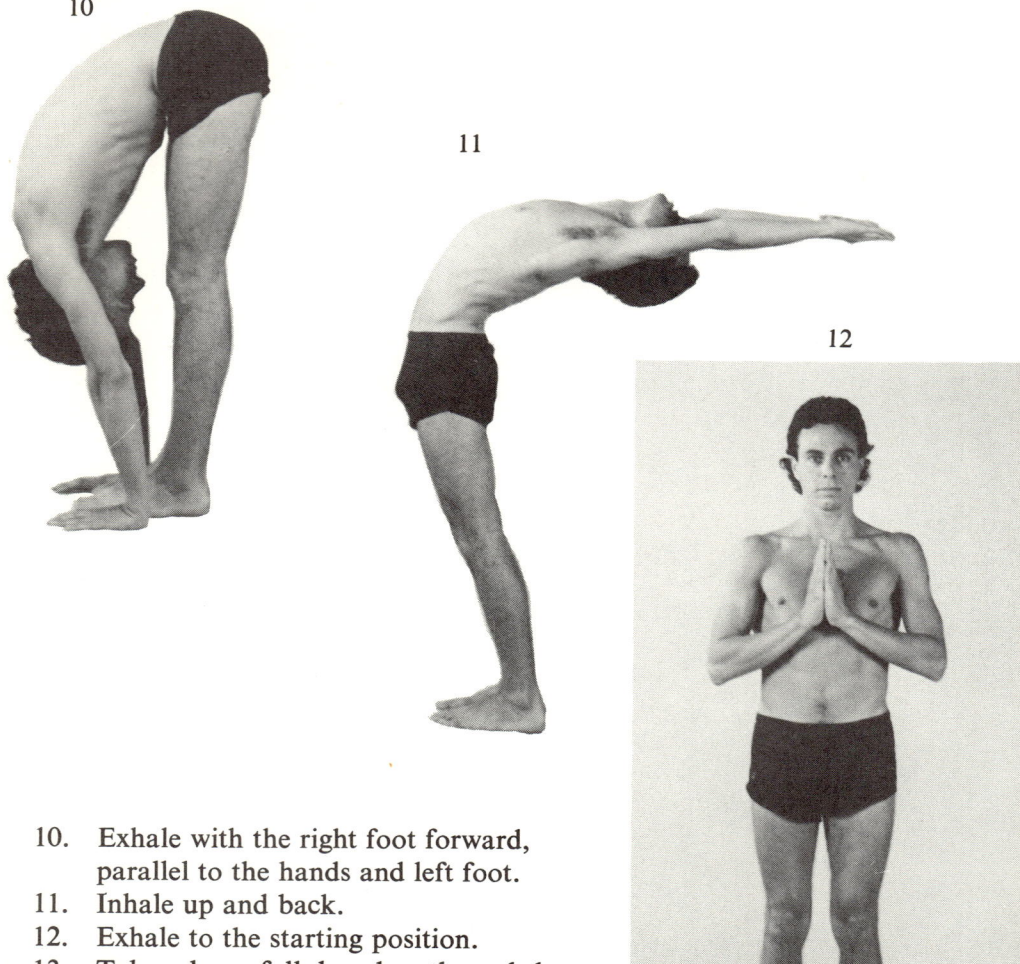

10. Exhale with the right foot forward, parallel to the hands and left foot.
11. Inhale up and back.
12. Exhale to the starting position.
13. Take a long, full deep breath, and then repeat all over again.

Note: As you repeat this series of postures, lead with the left leg for one round, then lead with the right leg for the next round.

The Rejuvenation Series

This series is a set of exercises also known as the Six Tibetans. Originally taken from a remote Himalayan monastery, the Six Tibetans are relatively easy to perform, but are profound for their ability to renew the body's natural life forces, inhibit the aging process, and endow the practitioner with boundless vitality.

By powerfully stimulating various nerve centers and glands within the body, the Six Tibetans promote a strong immune defense system, maintain keenly developed nerve transmission, and establish a balanced hormonal climate. In addition, the Six Tibetans tone and stretch the muscles, creating a stronger, more flexible body.

The morning is an excellent time to perform this series. At that time you will supercharge your system with vital life energy that will circulate through you all day long. You may also wish to practice the Six Tibetans again at night, before retiring. This enhances the quality of sleep, making it deeper and more refreshing.

The first five Tibetans are practiced for an optimal number of twenty-one times each. The final Tibetan is practiced only three times. You may need to work up to this number. In fact, almost all practitioners find that they need to build up to the maximum number over a period of a month or so. Take your time; as you go along, the Tibetans will be working for you. The effects that you will feel occur as the vital/psychic energies flow more strongly through you. According to the Yogis who developed this series, there is no need to exceed twenty-one repetitions for the exercises, as it is that number which produces the optimal effect.

Exercise #1
Stand up straight with the arms outstretched to the sides. The fingers are together, palms open and down. Now spin in a full circle in a clockwise direction. Repeat the spin twenty-one times without a break. When you are done, stand with the

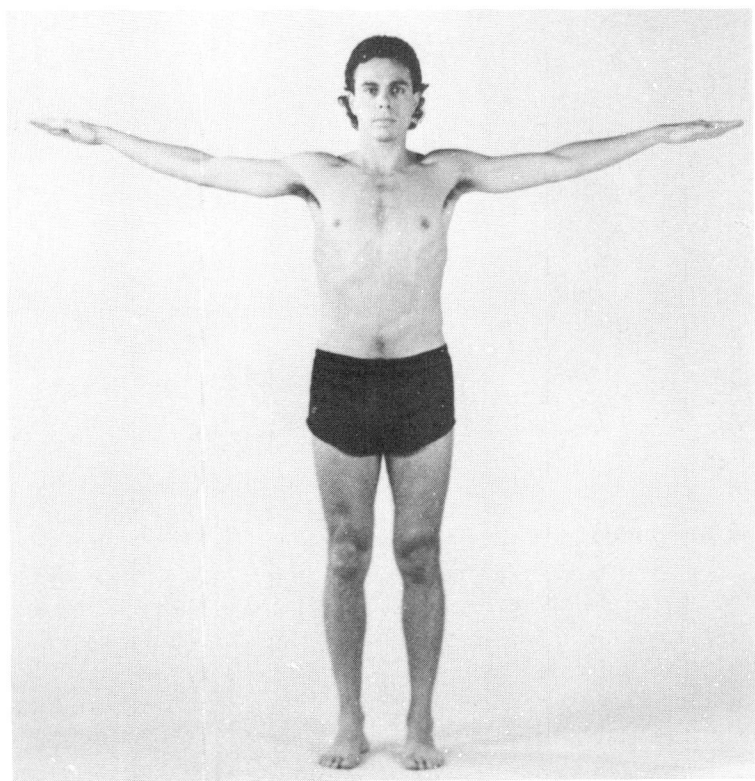

Exercise #1

hands on the hips and take two long, deep breaths, exhaling out the mouth. Take two breaths in this manner after each of the Tibetans.

Please note that the direction in which you spin is clockwise. If you were to turn your head to the right, you would spin in that direction. You may experience some dizziness when you first start to practice this. Don't do too much too quickly. With regular practice the dizziness will stop and the motion will be easy, even at high speeds.

Exercise #2
Lie on your back on a mat or rug. The legs are together and out straight, and the arms are by the sides with the palms flat on the floor. As you inhale, raise the legs up straight. The toes will be pointing toward the ceiling, but the lower back remains flat on the ground. As you bring the legs up, the head comes up also, with the chin tucked against the chest. This is all done in one smooth motion.

As you exhale, bring the legs and head down to the first position, with the body supine. Repeat the entire motion twenty-one times, inhaling as you bring the legs and head up, and exhaling as they come down.

Exercise #2

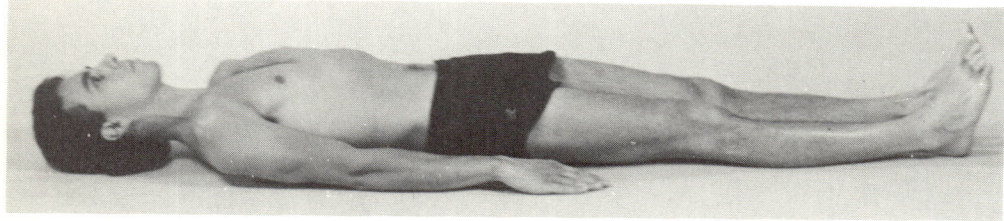

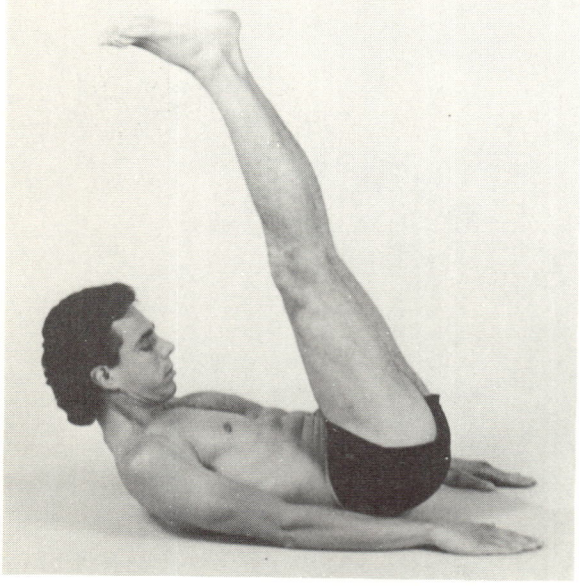

Exercise #3

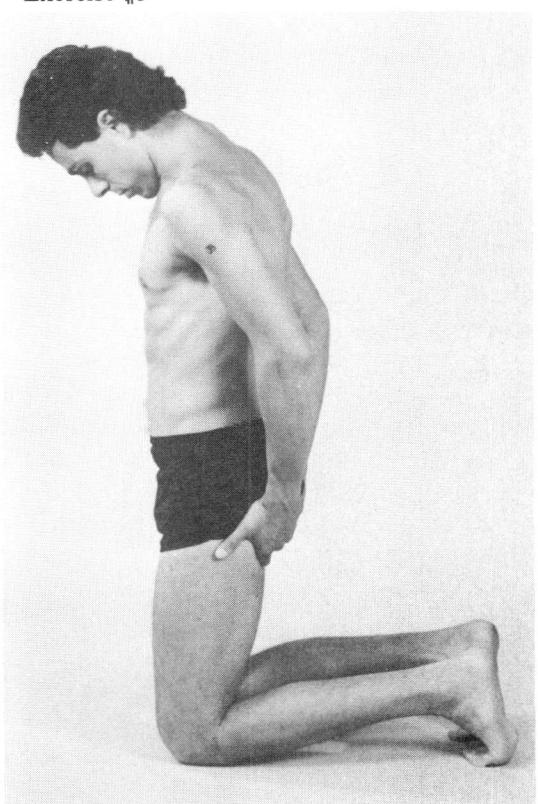

Exercise #3
Stand up on the knees and up on the balls of the feet. The knees are about four inches apart. The hands are placed with the palms flat against the backs of the thighs, just below the buttocks. The chin is tucked into the chest, though you are standing straight.

Inhale, and as you do, arch back from the waist, dropping the head back as far as it will go. Your hands will support you as you lean back. Then exhale, returning up and forward to the first position. Repeat the entire motion twenty-one times in a steady, unbroken rhythm.

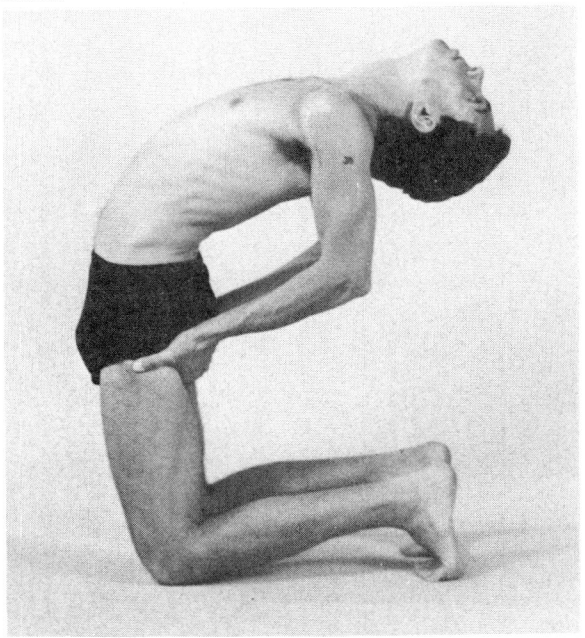

46/Yoga and Yogatherapy

Exercise #4

Sit up straight with the legs together and outstretched in front of you. The chin is tucked into the chest, and the arms are straight by the sides with the palms flat against the floor beside your hips. Placement of the hands is particularly important; they should be exactly beside the hips.

Inhale and raise the hips, bending the knees up, bringing the soles of the feet flat to the floor. You will come into a position in which the body is parallel to the floor while the arms and legs are in a vertical position. The head is dropped all the way back. Then exhale and come back down to the original position.

Repeat the motion twenty-one times in a steady rhythm. Please note that in this exercise the feet do not slide; they stay in the same place. The arms do not bend at all; you merely pivot on the shoulders.

Exercise #4

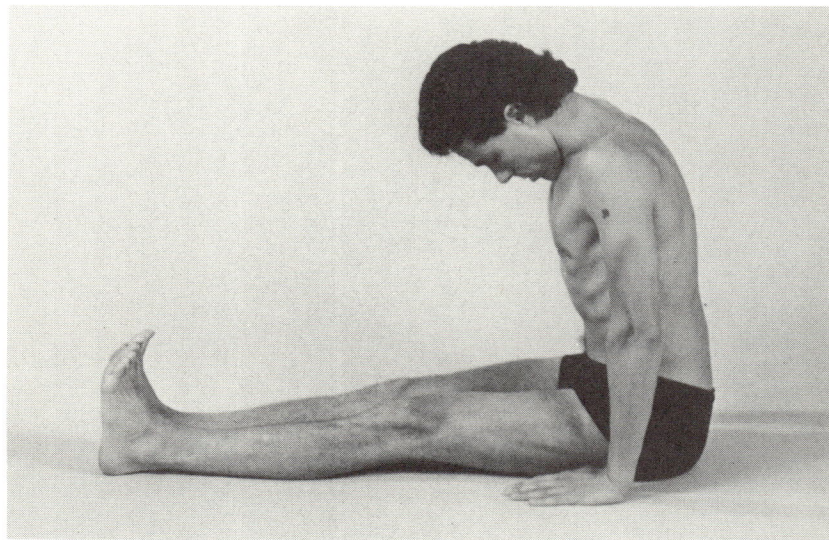
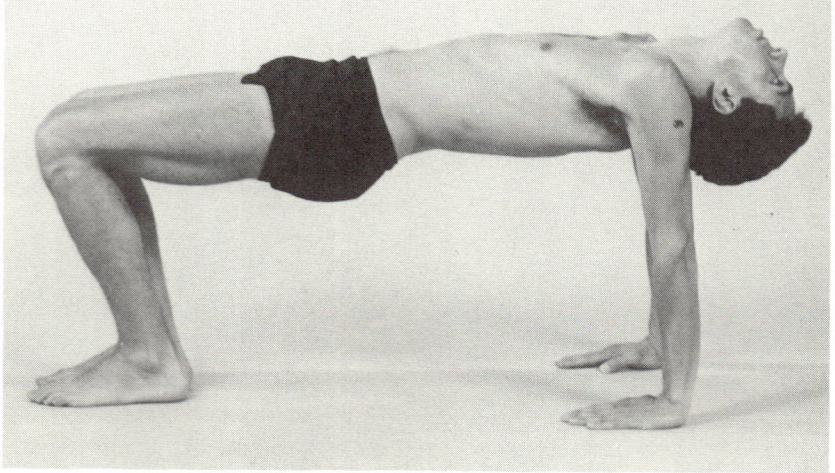

Exercise #5

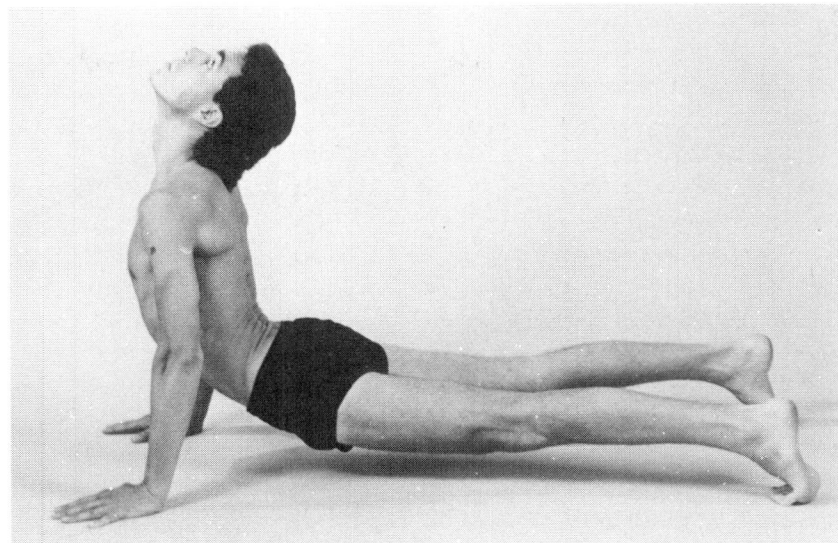

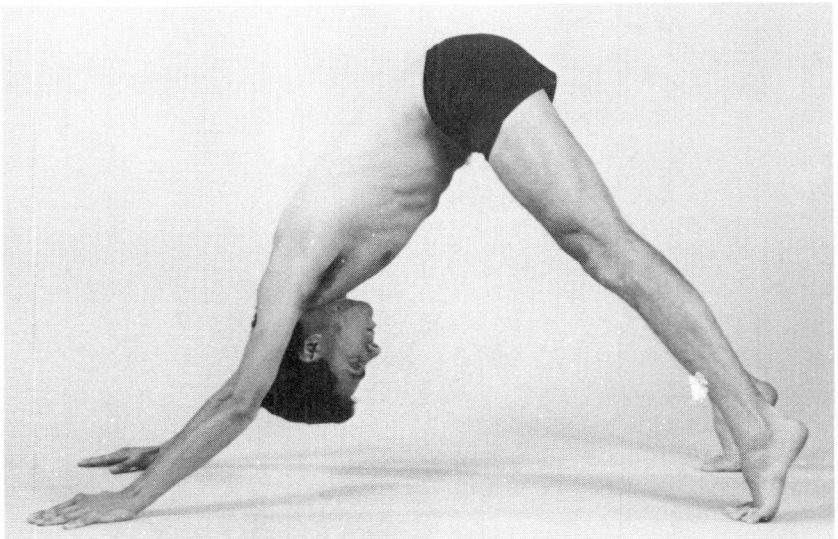

Exercise #5
Start out on the hands and the balls of the feet, as though preparing to do push-ups. The hands are about two feet apart, as are the feet. Keeping the arms and legs perfectly straight, inhale as you raise the buttocks toward the sky, bringing your body into a perfect triangle. The chin is tucked into the chest in this position. Then exhale down to the starting position, with the head back as you sag down.

Your body should be off the ground or just barely touching. Repeat the entire motion twenty-one times, and then rest on your back for a couple of minutes before performing the Sixth Tibetan.

Exercise #6

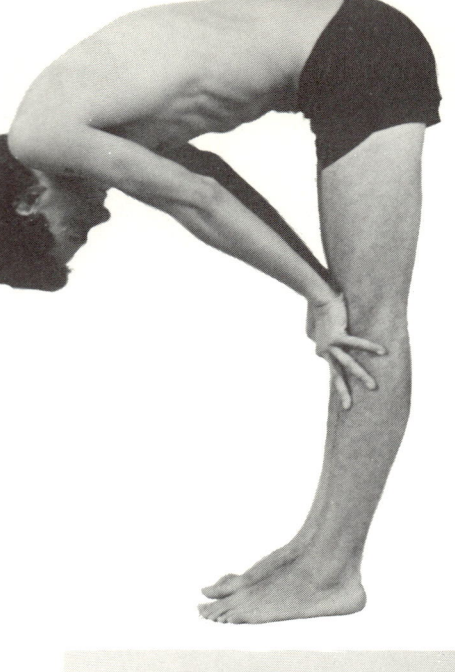

Exercise #6
Stand up straight with the hands on the hips. The feet are about four inches apart. In this position take a long, deep breath. Then exhale, and as you do, bend forward, leaning on the knees with your hands.

In this position squeeze out all the breath, so that the abdomen is pulled in tightly. Then, while holding the breath out, come back up to a standing position again, with the hands on the hips. In this position, with the abdomen pulled in tightly, hold your breath out for as long as is comfortable. Then take a deep breath and relax.

Repeat this technique a maximum of three times. Finish with two deep breaths with the hands on the hips, as with the other five Tibetans. Then relax on your back for a couple of minutes.

The Squat

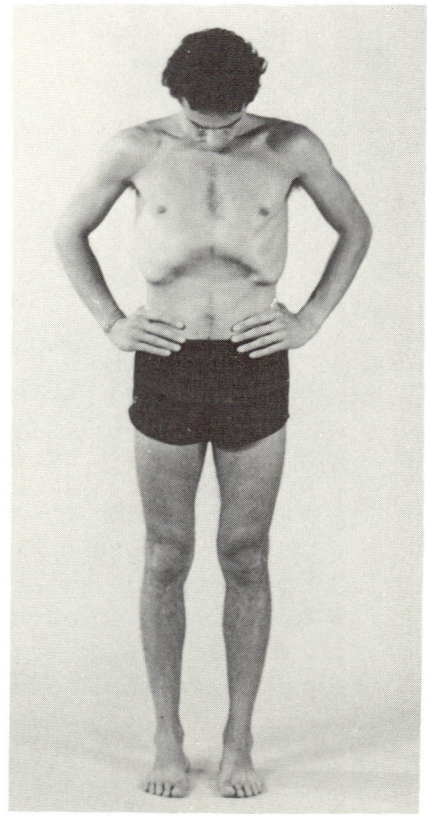

Stand with the feet approximately shoulder's width apart. Bend the knees, lowering the buttocks as far as possible. The arms rest between the knees, and the heels are flat on the floor. This may be difficult at first, and you may feel that if you flatten your heels on the floor, you will lose your balance. Most often this is not the case. However, initially you may wish to hold onto a table leg or post until you are comfortable in the position.

Interlock the fingers and gently rock back

The Squat

The Wide Squat

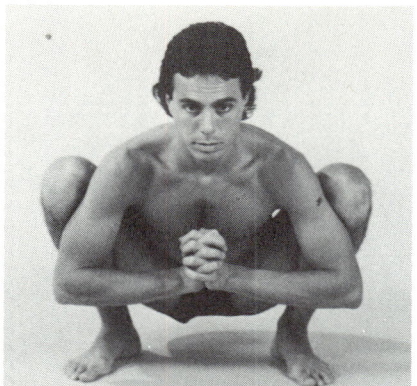
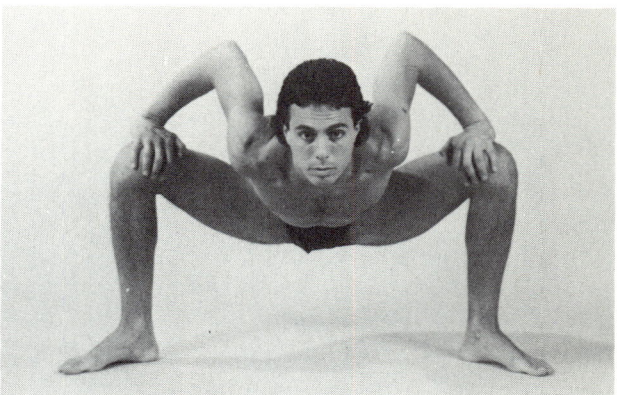

Palm Pose

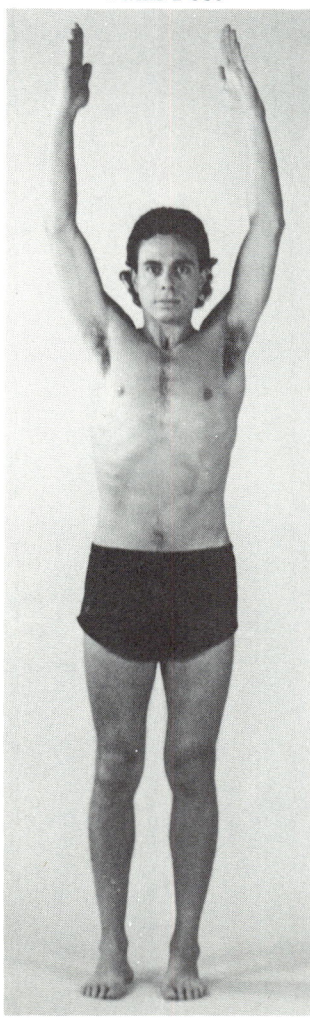

and forth. Start out doing this for just a minute or so, and build up to several minutes.

Benefits: Stretches the hips, breaks up tension in the pelvis, frees blocked sexual energy, stretches the lower spine, soothes the nervous system, is an excellent position in which to move the bowels.

The Wide Squat

Stand with the feet almost twice your shoulder's width apart. The feet are flat on the floor and are partially turned out to the sides. With your hands on your knees, lower your buttocks as far as you can. There will be muscular resistance in the hips and crotch. When you encounter this resistance, gently bounce down a little bit at a time. Do this for a half minute or so, and come up. Work at this until you can bounce comfortably in the position for two minutes.

Benefits: Stretches the hips, breaks up tension in the pelvis, strengthens the legs, increases circulation to the crotch area.

Palm Pose

Stand with the feet together, the legs straight, and the body upright, with the arms upstretched straight with

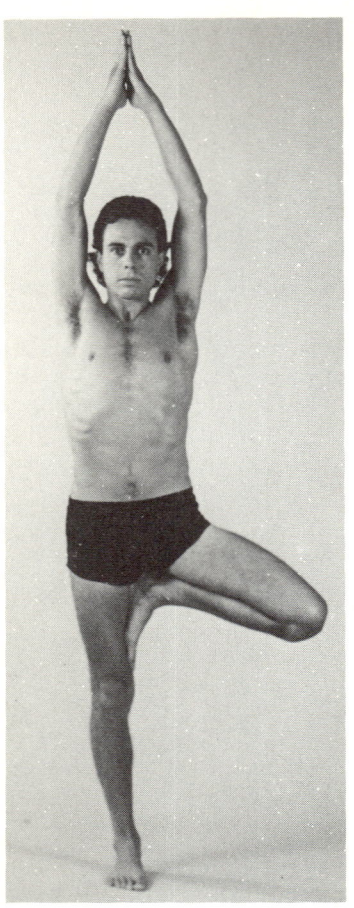

the fingers together and the palms facing each other. Stretch as high up as you can. In this position, breathe long and deep, for one minute or more.

Benefits: Strengthens and tones the legs, stretches the spine, opens the shoulder joints, opens up the lungs, stimulates intestinal activity, improves posture.

One Legged Pose

Stand with your left leg straight and the left foot flat on the floor. Tuck the heel of your right foot into your crotch, with the sole flat against the left inner thigh. Straighten your body upright, stretching your arms up as high as possible with the palms together. Breathe long and deep for a minute or more. Switch legs and repeat.

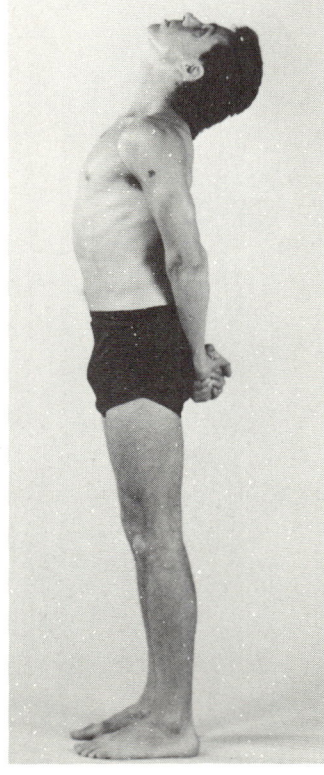

Neck Pose

One Legged Pose

Benefits: Develops balance, strengthens and tones legs, increases flexibility of the knees, stretches the spine, opens the shoulder joints, opens up the lungs, stimulates intestinal activity, improves posture.

Neck Pose

Standing straight with the arms by the sides, inhale and stretch the head up and back, as far as you can. Exhale, and bring the head forward and down, tucking the chin into the chest. Breathe and move slowly, repeating the motion ten or more times.

Benefits: Stretches and strengthens the neck, opens up the bronchial passages, and stimulates circulation to the thyroid.

Triangle Pose

Stand with the feet almost twice your shoulder's width apart, with the arms outstretched to the sides, palms down. Inhale in this upright position. Then exhale, as you twist, rotate and turn from the lower waist and hips, bringing your left hand down to your right foot, with your head turned up and right. Then inhale back up to the upright position, and exhale down to the other side. Repeat on each side eight times or more, stretching and rotating more each time you do.

Benefits: Increases spinal flexibility, stretches the backs of the legs, enhances posture, increases circulation to the internal organs, energizes the spinal nerves, strengthens the legs, enhances intestinal activity.

Triangle Pose

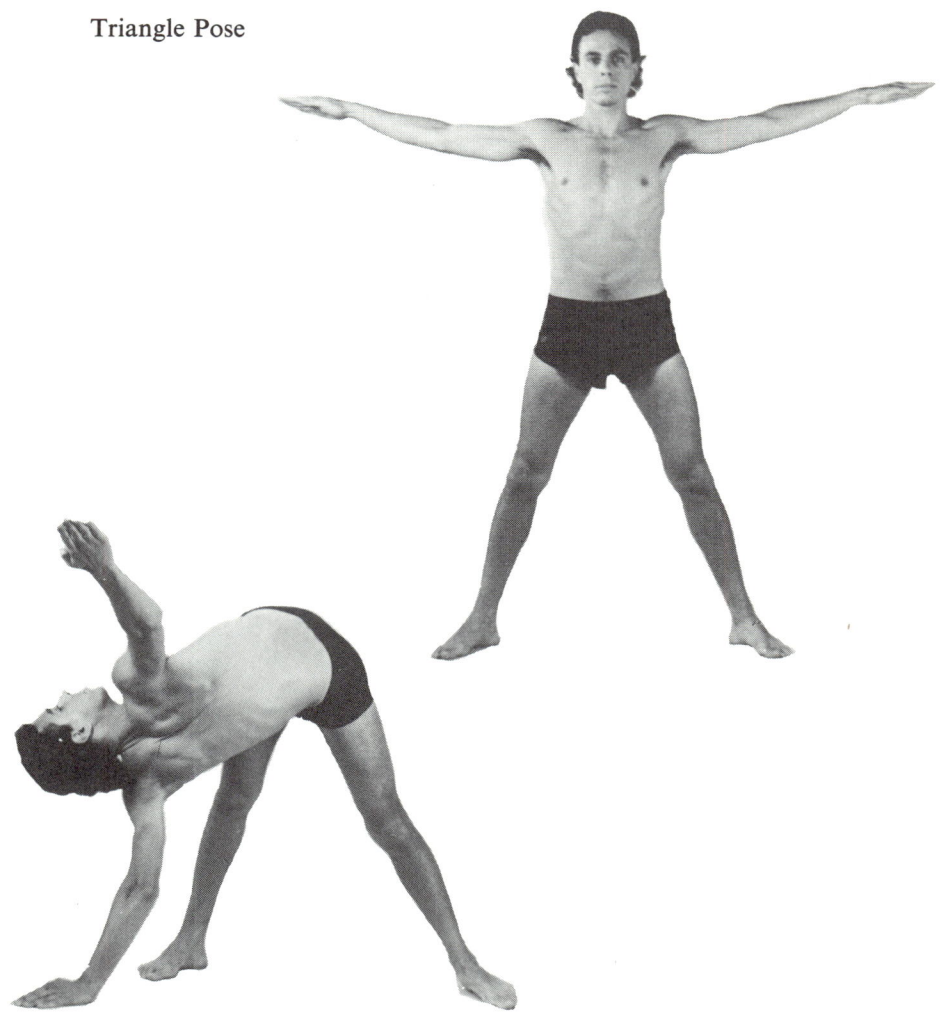

Side Stretch

Stand with the feet almost twice your shoulder's width apart, standing up straight. Stretch directly to the right, sliding your right hand down your right leg as far as you can, while you stretch your left arm up over your head and to the right. Exhale as you stretch to the side. Inhale up, and exhale to the left side. Repeat eight times or more.

Benefits: Stretches the spine, opens up the rib cage, opens up the lungs, improves posture, enhances circulation to the kidneys and lower internal organs.

Side Stretch

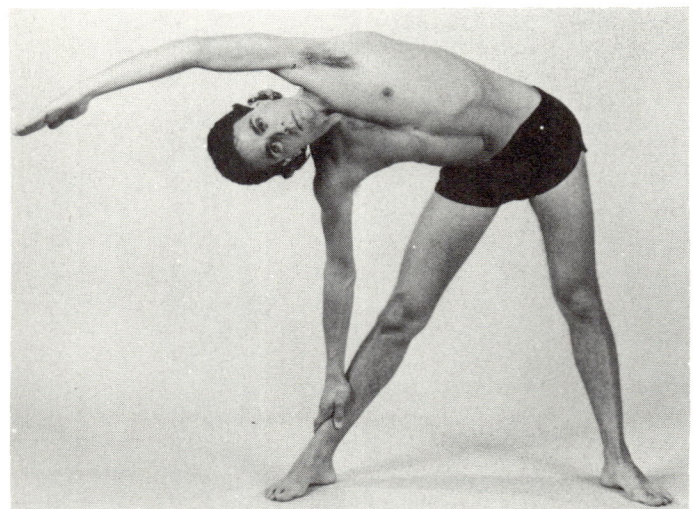

Standing Leg Stretch

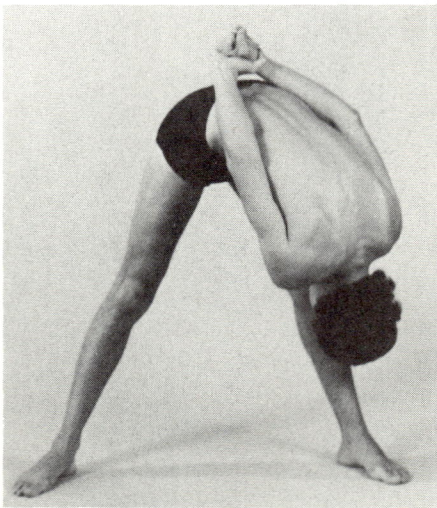

Standing Leg Stretch

Stand with the feet almost twice your shoulder's width apart, with your body upright. Your hands are clasped behind your back. Inhale as you stand up straight, and then exhale, stretching down over one leg, touching your head to your knee. Inhale up, and repeat on the other side. Repeat on each side eight times or more, stretching as far down as you can each time.

Benefits: Stretches out the backs of the legs, enhances lower spinal flexibility, increases circulation to the head, stimulates digestive activity.

Palm to Floor Pose

Stand with the feet just a few inches apart, with the legs straight and the body upright. The arms are stretched upright as far as you can. Inhale in this upright position, and exhale, stretching down as far as you can, bringing the hands to the floor, keeping the legs straight. Inhale up straight again. Repeat ten or more times.

Once you have become very flexible in this position, hold yourself in the down position, with the legs straight and the head down, with the palms flat on the floor. In this posture, breathe slowly and evenly for a minute or more.

Benefits: Stretches the backs of the legs, enhances spinal flexibility, improves overall circulation, stimulates digestive activity, energizes the spinal nerves.

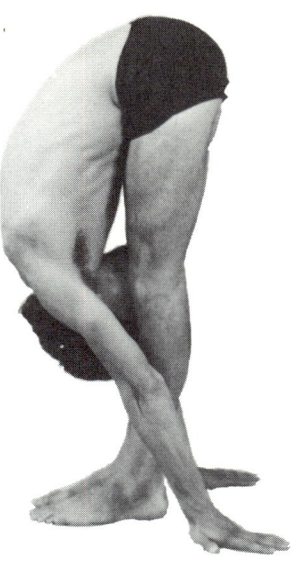

Palm to Floor Pose

Standing Back Stretch

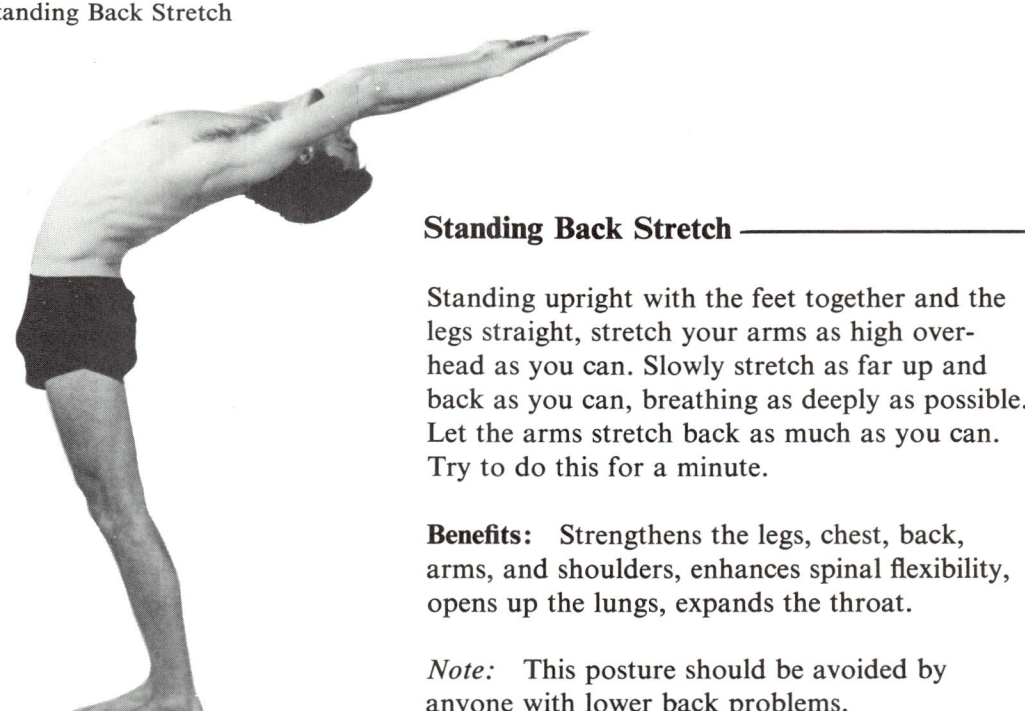

Standing Back Stretch

Standing upright with the feet together and the legs straight, stretch your arms as high overhead as you can. Slowly stretch as far up and back as you can, breathing as deeply as possible. Let the arms stretch back as much as you can. Try to do this for a minute.

Benefits: Strengthens the legs, chest, back, arms, and shoulders, enhances spinal flexibility, opens up the lungs, expands the throat.

Note: This posture should be avoided by anyone with lower back problems.

Forward Knee Pose

Place one foot flat on the ground with your hands to each side of the foot, fingertips resting on the ground. Extend your other leg as far back as you can, stretching your shoulders up and back, with your chin stretching up. In this position, breathe gently and evenly, allowing the muscles in your body to stretch and relax as you breathe. Do this for a minute or more on each side.

Benefits: Stretches out the hips and crotch, improves posture, opens up the throat.

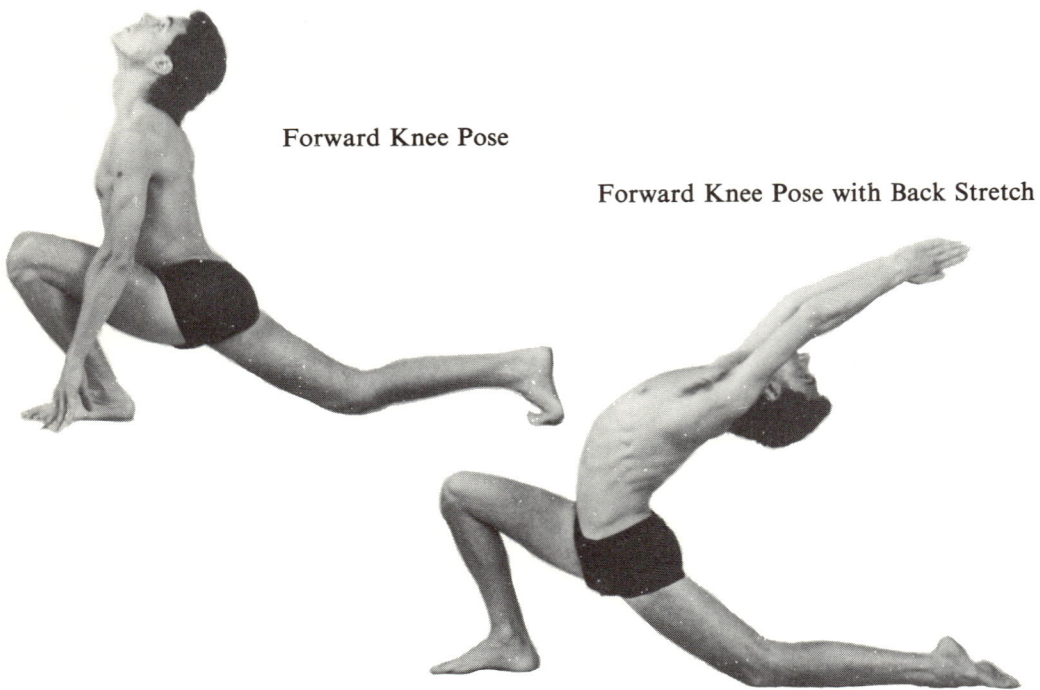

Forward Knee Pose

Forward Knee Pose with Back Stretch

Forward Knee Pose with Back Stretch

Place one foot flat on the ground with the knee bent, and the other leg stretched out as far as possible behind you, with the instep flat on the ground. With your palms together, stretch your arms up and back, arching your back as far as possible as you stretch. In this position, breathe long and deep. Try to do this for a minute.

Benefits: Stretches out the hips and crotch, strenghtens the back and chest, opens up the throat and lungs, improves posture, strengthens legs.

Note: This posture should be avoided by anyone with lower back problems.

Forward Knee/Palm Pose

Stand with your right foot flat on the floor, with the right knee bent at a right angle. Extend your left leg straight back, keeping it straight, with the left foot flat on the floor, pointing to the left. With the palms of the hands together, extend your arms as high overhead as you can, with your head back, as you look up at the hands. Breathe gently and steadily. Try to hold the position for a minute or more. Switch sides.

Benefits: Strengthens the legs, back, and chest, stretches open the ribs, opens the throat and lungs, strengthens the neck, improves posture, energizes the spinal nerves.

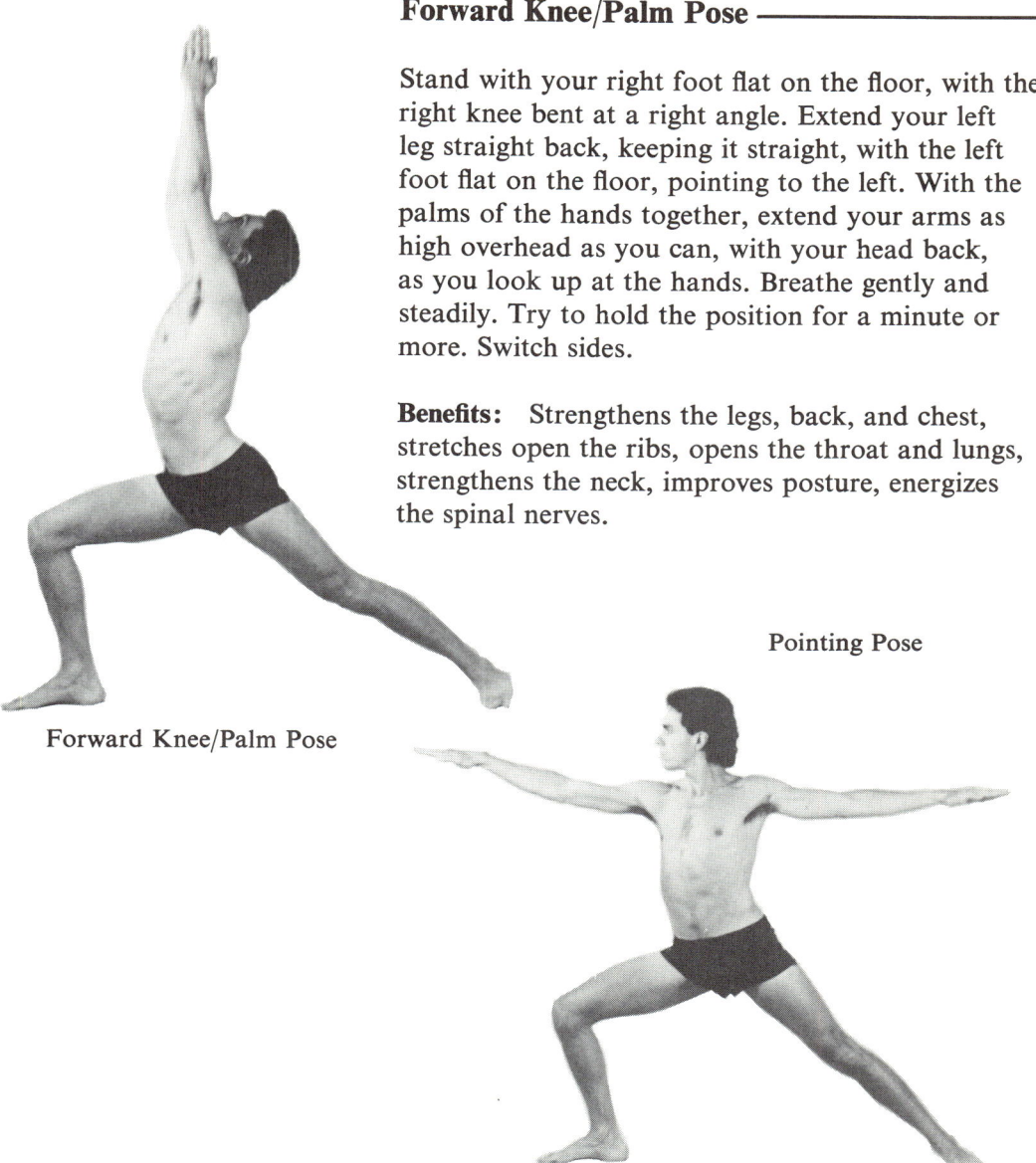

Forward Knee/Palm Pose

Pointing Pose

Pointing Pose

Stand with your right foot flat on the floor, with the right knee bent at a right angle. Extend your left leg straight back, keeping it straight, with the left foot flat on the floor, pointing to the left. Extend your arms straight out to the sides, with your right arm extended over your right leg, and your left arm extended over your left leg. Your head is turned to the right. Breathe long and deep for a minute or more, then switch sides.

Benefits: Strengthens the legs, improves posture, strengthens the arms and shoulders.

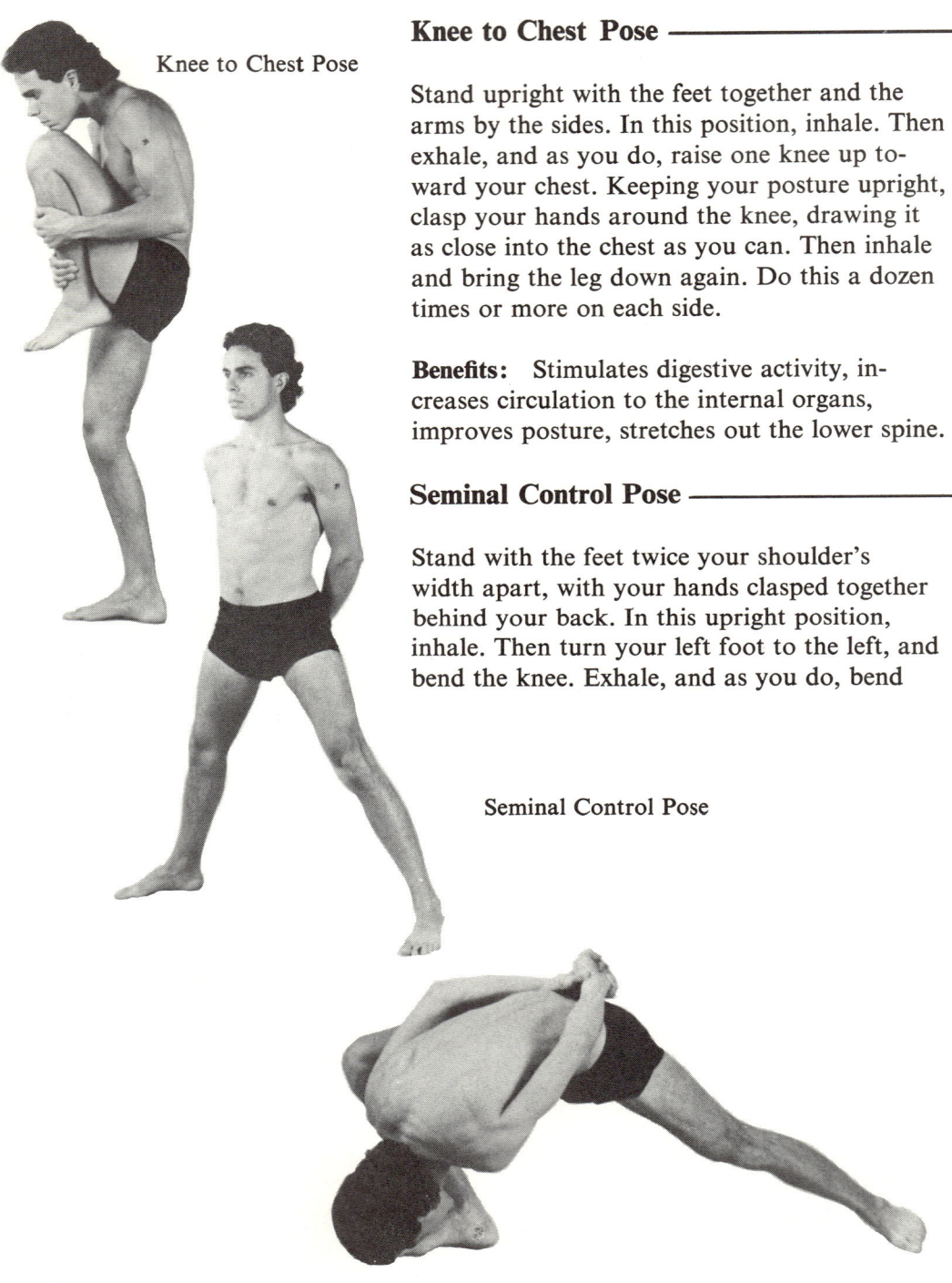

Knee to Chest Pose

Seminal Control Pose

Knee to Chest Pose

Stand upright with the feet together and the arms by the sides. In this position, inhale. Then exhale, and as you do, raise one knee up toward your chest. Keeping your posture upright, clasp your hands around the knee, drawing it as close into the chest as you can. Then inhale and bring the leg down again. Do this a dozen times or more on each side.

Benefits: Stimulates digestive activity, increases circulation to the internal organs, improves posture, stretches out the lower spine.

Seminal Control Pose

Stand with the feet twice your shoulder's width apart, with your hands clasped together behind your back. In this upright position, inhale. Then turn your left foot to the left, and bend the knee. Exhale, and as you do, bend down, bringing your head toward your left foot. You will need to get your leg out of the way as your chest moves downward. This is done by moving the knee to the left. The goal is to stretch down far enough to touch the toes with your nose. Then inhale upright again, bringing the left foot back to its original position. Then repeat the motion on the right side. Repeat this on each side ten or more times.

Benefits: Stretches out the crotch, strengthens the inner thighs, and acts specifically to give men control over ejaculation.

Supine Knee to Chest Pose

Lie on your back, with the legs straight out. Draw one knee close to the chest, with the hands clasped around the knee. The breath is normal and relaxed. Hold this position for a minute or more, then switch legs.

Benefits: Helps to eliminate intestinal gas, relieves lower back tension, stimulates circulation to the abdominal organs.

Supine Knee to Chest Pose

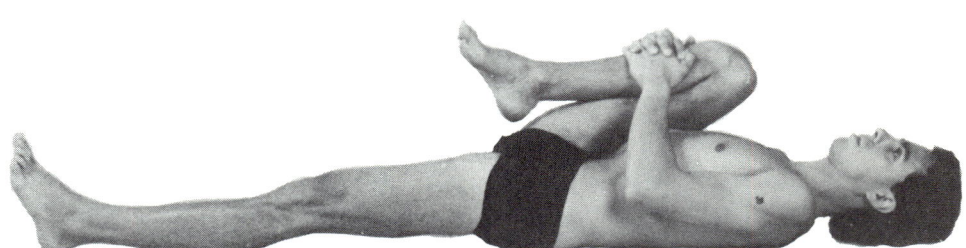

Wind Eliminating Pose

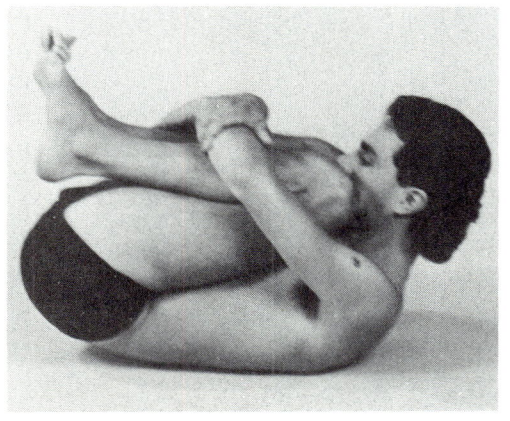

Wind Eliminating Pose

Lie on your back with both knees drawn to your chest, with the hands clasped around them. Bring your head up, with your nose tucked between the knees. Breathe normally in this position for a minute or more.

Benefits: Aids in elimination of intestinal gas, stimulates intestinal motion, relieves lower spinal tension, stretches the entire spine.

Moving Knees to Chest Pose

Lying on your back with your arms by your sides, draw your knees to your chest as you exhale. As you inhale, extend your legs out straight, with the feet about six inches off the ground. Keep repeating the motion and breathing pattern in a steady rhythm, about twenty or more times. Keep the lower back pressed against the ground throughout the exercise.

Benefits: Aids in elimination of intestinal gas, stimulates intestinal activity, strengthens the abdomen and the lower back, improves posture.

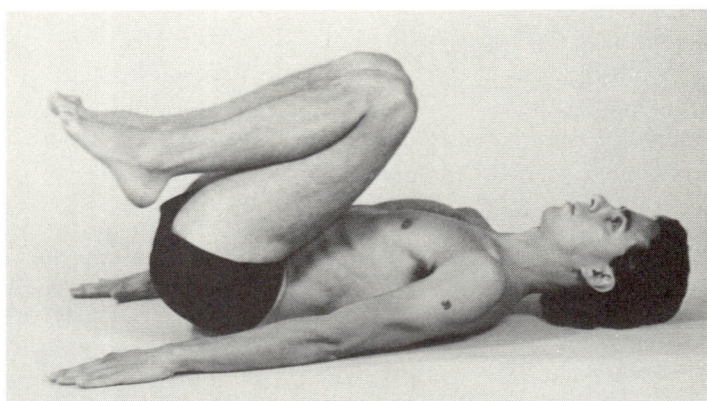

Moving Knees to Chest Pose

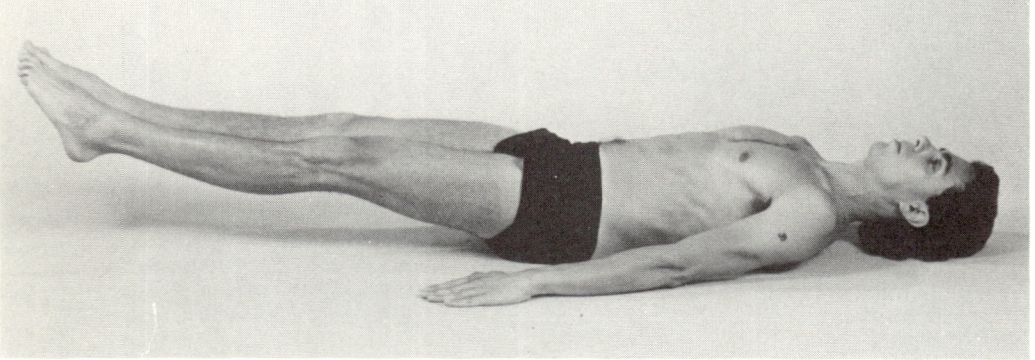

Inverted Leg Pose

Lie on your back with your arms by your sides, and the legs together pointing straight up toward the sky. The toes are pointed up. The breath is normal. Hold this position for a minute or longer, making sure to keep the lower spine pressed firmly against the ground the entire time.

Inverted Leg Pose

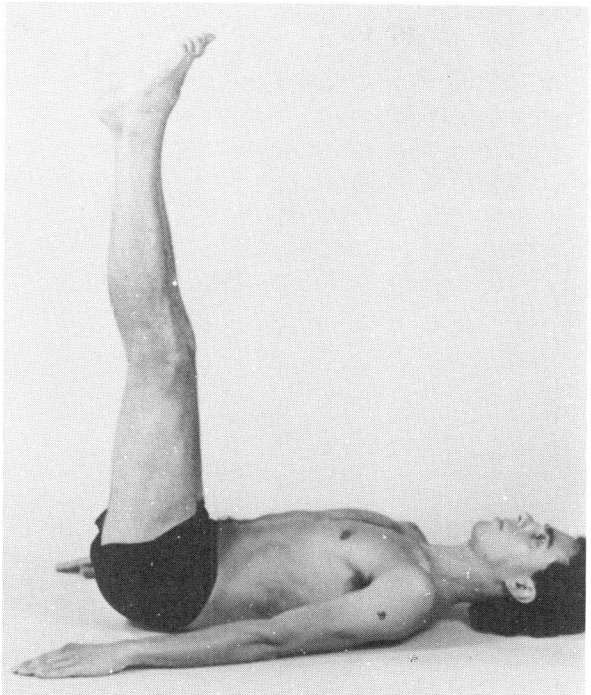

Benefits: Enhances circulation to the lower abdomen, strengthens the lower spine, relieves circulatory pressure from the legs, enhances intestinal activity.

Celibate Pose

Sit on the ground with the buttocks between the feet, leaning on your elbows. Lower yourself until your back is also on the ground. Once in this position, extend your arms straight out behind you, with the palms facing upward. In this position, breathe long and deep, for a minute or longer.

Benefits: Stretches out the knees and ankles, improves circulation to the pelvis and sex organs, stimulates digestion, stretches out the chest.

Celibate Pose

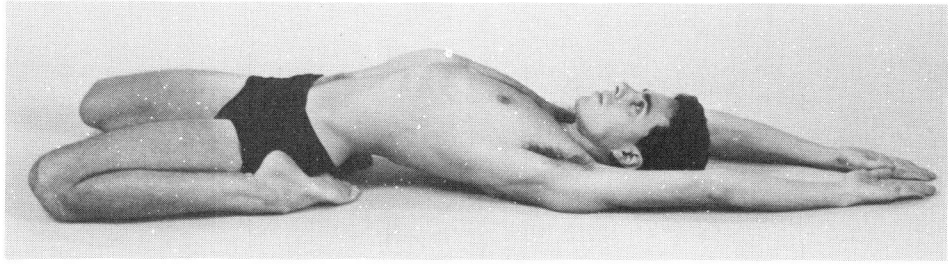

Supine Spinal Twist

Lie on your back with your legs together pointing straight upward, and your arms extended out to the sides with the palms up. Inhale in this position. Exhale, and as you do, stretch your legs over to one side, bringing them all the way down to the ground, keeping the shoulders and arms firmly planted on the ground. The rotation is all in the lower and middle spine. Then inhale back up straight. Repeat on each side twenty times or more.

Benefits: Increases intestinal activity, improves digestion, increases spinal flexibility, improves posture, strengthens the abdomen and lower back.

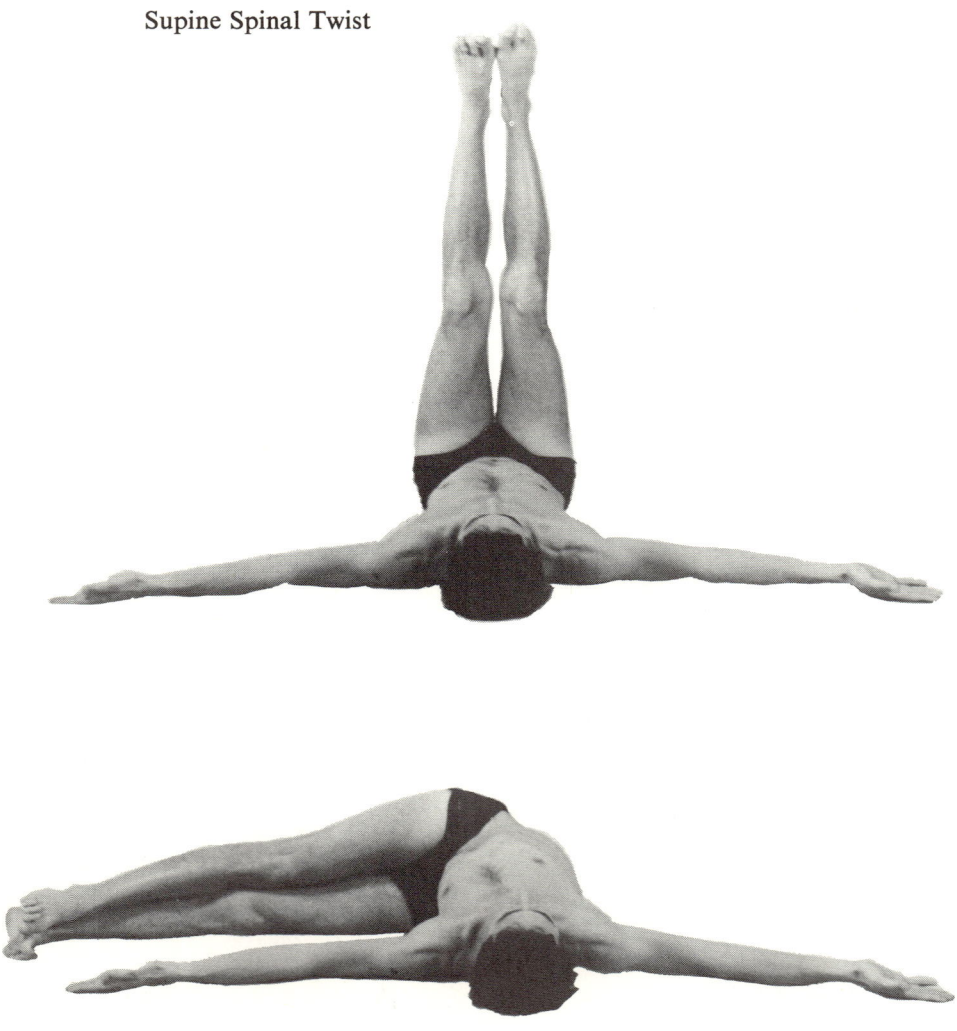

Supine Spinal Twist

Crotch Stretch

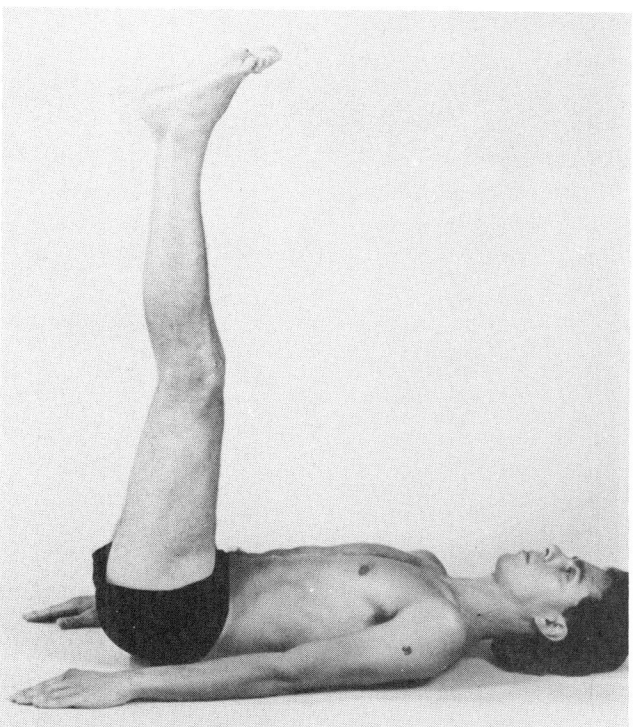

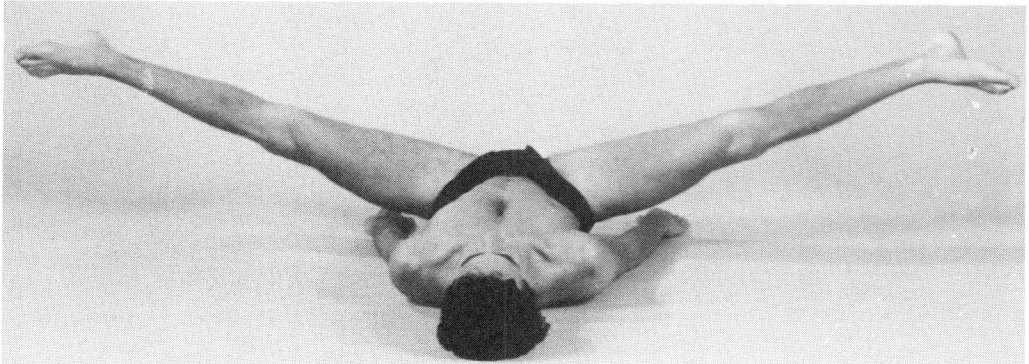

Crotch Stretch

Lie on your back with the legs extended straight upward, and the arms by your sides. The toes are pointing up, and the back is flat against the ground. As you inhale, stretch the legs wide apart, keeping them straight. Exhale, bringing the legs together again. Do this twenty times in a steady rhythm.

Benefits: Loosens the crotch and hips, and stimulates the lower spinal nerves.

Pelvic Pose

Lie on your back, with the knees up and the soles of your feet flat on the ground, tucked close to the buttocks. The feet are about fifteen inches apart, with the hands firmly holding the ankles. As you inhale, stretch your hips up toward the sky, arching your spine forward. As you exhale, come back down to the first position. Repeat this twenty times in a steady rhythm, each time stretching a little bit further.

Benefits: Loosens the spine, stimulates the sex organs, opens up the pelvis, strengthens the thighs, improves posture.

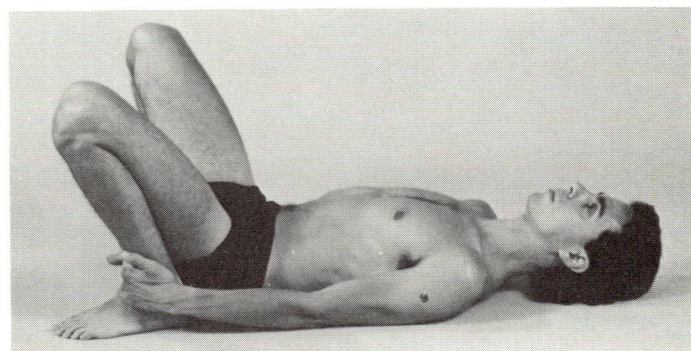

Pelvic Pose

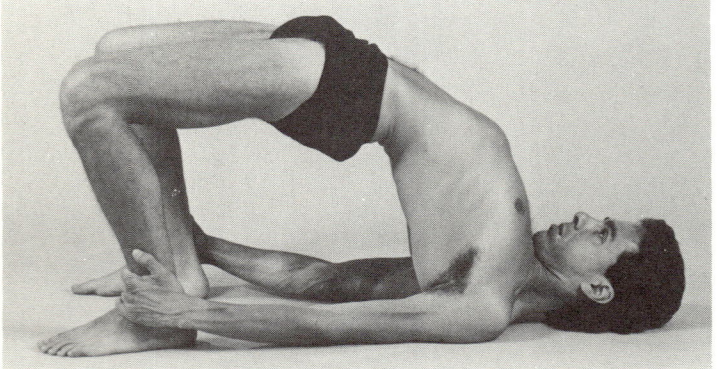

Easy Pose

Sit down with the legs folded comfortably, with the hands resting on the knees. Keep your trunk upright, with the lower spine tucked slightly forward. In this position, breathe normally for several minutes. Get used to sitting in this position for longer periods of time.

Benefits: Improves posture, enhances circulation of energy throughout the nervous system, enables the body to relax while upright, improves flexibility of the legs.

Easy Pose

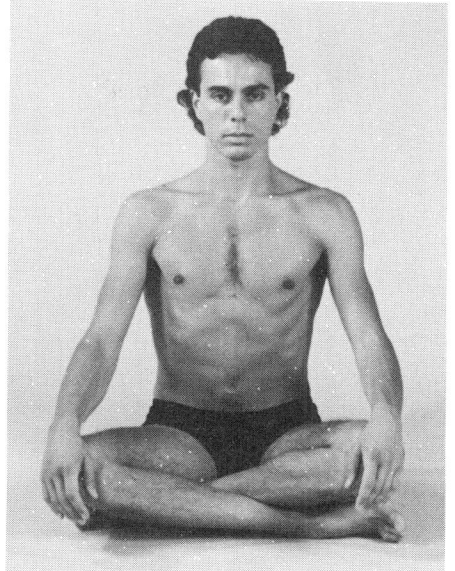

Rock Pose

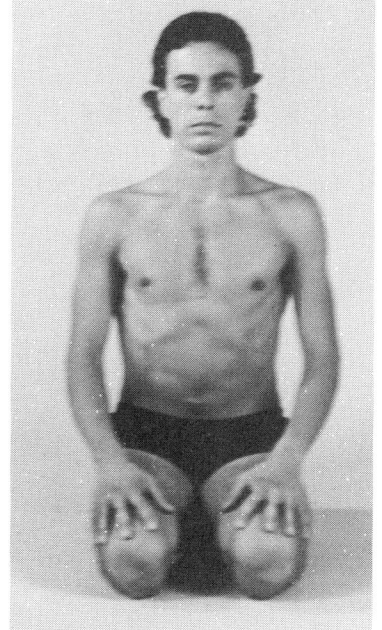

Rock Pose

Sit on the knees, sitting back on the heels, with the feet together. The hands are resting on the thighs, and the trunk is upright.

Benefits: Enhances digestion, strengthens the back, improves posture.

Hero Pose

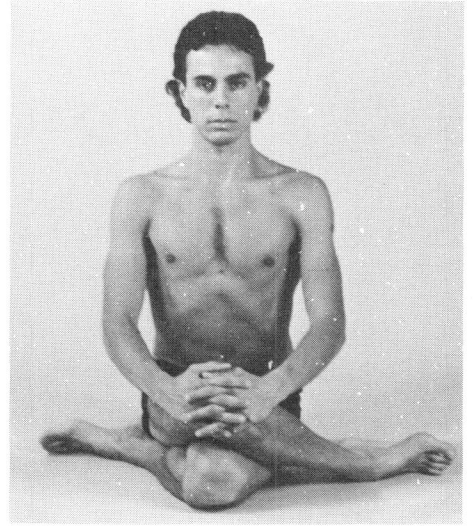

Hero Pose

Sitting on the ground, tuck your left heel tightly into the right buttock. Place your right leg over your left, tucking the heel close to the left buttock. Sit up as straight as possible. Breathe normally for a couple of minutes, then switch legs and repeat.

Benefits: Stimulates the sex organs, energizes the lower spinal nerves, strengthens the lower back, improves posture.

Cow Head Pose

Sitting on the ground, tuck your left heel tightly into the right buttock. Place your right leg over your left, tucking the heel close to the left buttock. Sit up as straight as possible. Raise the left arm and bend it from the elbow, turning it back and slightly downward. Turn the right arm behind you, and bend it up from the elbow, trying to catch the fingers of your left hand. Try to stretch the left elbow upward as high as possible. In this position, breathe long and deep for a minute or two. Then switch arms and legs and repeat.

Benefits: Stimulates the sex organs, energizes the spinal nerves, strengthens the back, stretches the arms, improves posture, opens the rib cage.

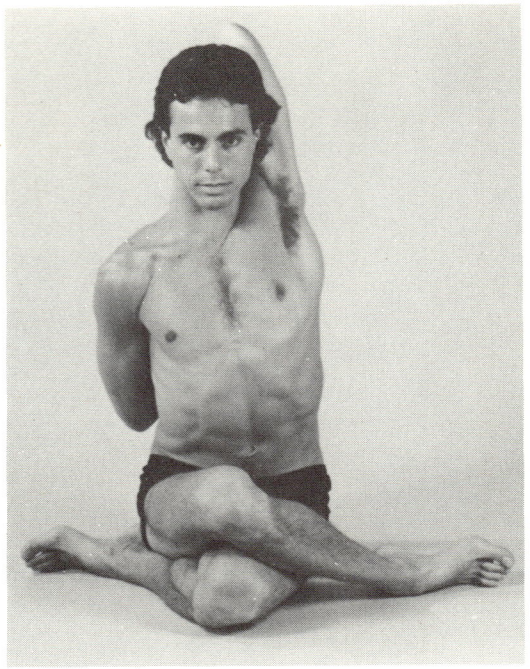
Cow Head Pose

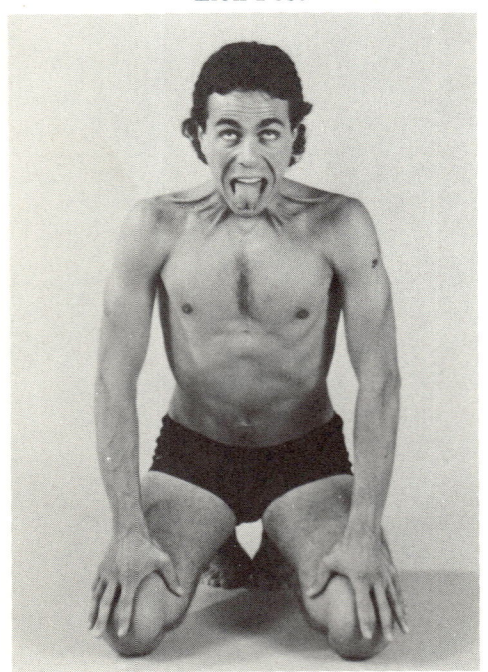
Lion Pose

Lion Pose

Sit on the knees, resting back on the heels of the feet, with the balls of the feet resting on the floor. The hands are on the knees, and the knees are about six inches apart. Open the mouth as wide as possible, and stretch your tongue out as far as you can. Inhale and exhale deeply through the mouth six to ten times.

Benefits: Reduces tension in the jaw muscles, improves vocal tone, opens the throat, tones facial muscles, stimulates circulation to the face, improves the sense of taste.

Lotus Pose

Sitting upright on the ground, tuck the outer edge of your left foot into the crease of your right hip and inner thigh. Pull your right foot up over your left leg, tucking the outer edge of the right foot into the crease of your left hip and inner thigh. The hands are resting on the knees, with the tips of the thumbs and forefingers touching. The spine is erect, and the breath is normal and even. This posture may be held for hours at a time. Initially, try to maintain Lotus pose for a couple of minutes. Gradually increase the time. This is the ideal pose for meditation.

Benefits: Circulates life energy throughout the entire nervous system, improves posture, strengthens the lower back, improves flexibility of the legs, has a stabilizing effect upon all bodily functions.

Lotus Spinal Stretch

Sitting in Lotus Pose, interlock the fingers, and extend the arms as high upward as possible, with the palms facing the sky. In this position, breathe long and deep for a couple of minutes.

Benefits: Increases the flow of life energy throughout the entire nervous system, strengthens the back, improves posture, increases circulation to the head, stretches the arms, clears the mind, opens the lungs.

Lotus Pose

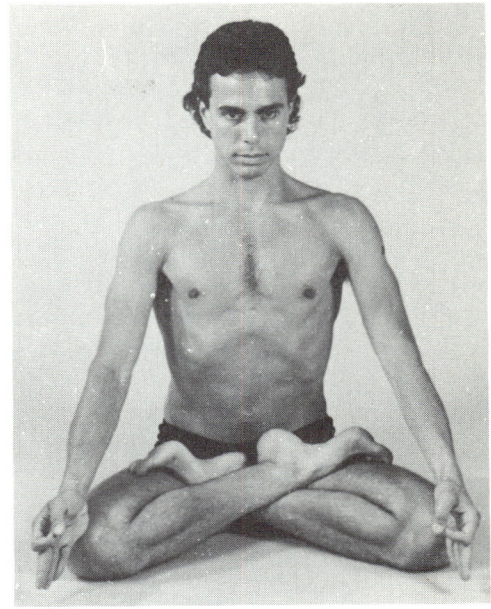

Lotus Spinal Stretch

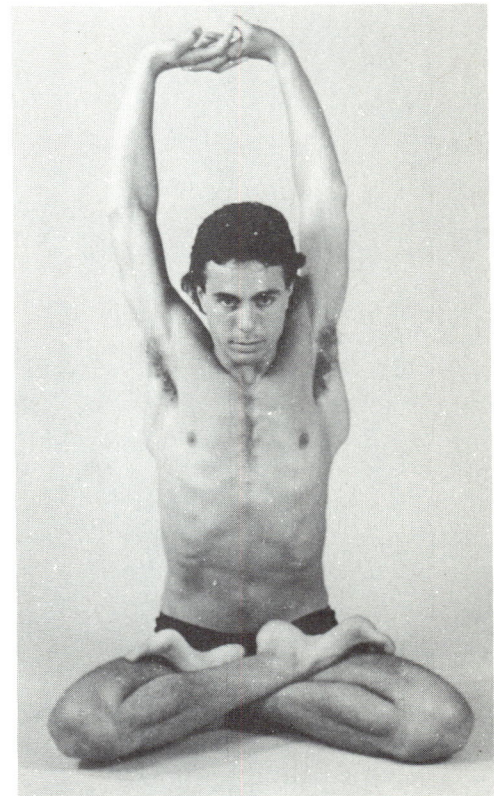

Butterfly Pose

Sitting with the soles of the feet together, draw the feet as close in to the crotch as possible. Hold the feet with your hands and gently bounce the knees.

After you have bounced the knees a few times, inhale with the spine upright, and then exhale forward, bringing your head as close to the ground as possible. The stretch is from the hips. Stretch up and down with the breath twenty times.

Benefits: Opens the pelvis, stretches the hip joints, frees blocked energy, stimulates sexual nerves, loosens the lower spine, improves posture.

Butterfly Pose

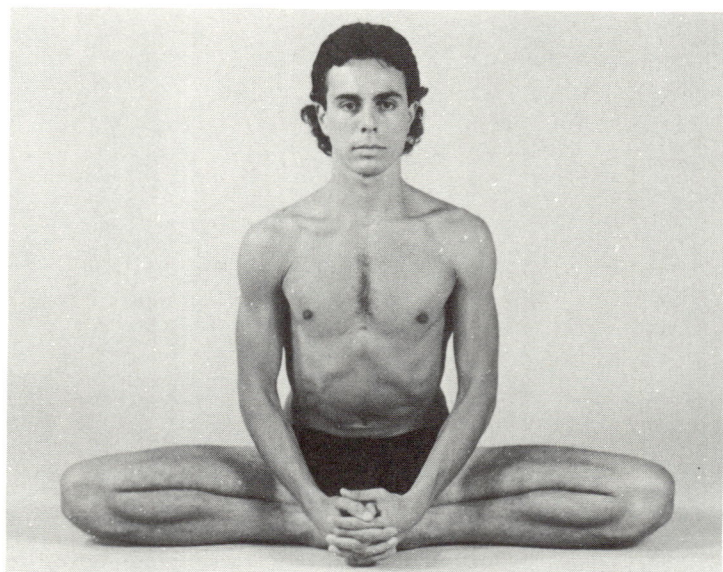

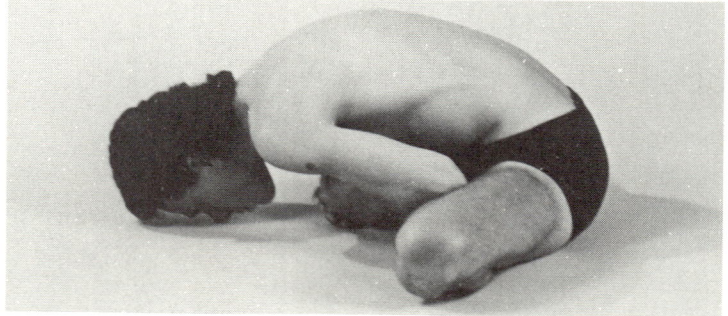

Leg Splits

Sit with the legs stretched as wide apart as possible. Inhale in the upright position, with your trunk up straight. Exhale, stretching down over one leg, reaching for the foot with both hands. Inhale up again, and stretch down over the other leg.

Repeat a dozen times or so. Then inhale in the upright position, and exhale straight down, stretching the chest down to the ground. Repeat this stretch several times, then rest for a moment in the down position, breathing normally.

Benefits: Stretches out the backs of the legs, the hips, pelvis, and lower spine, and improves circulation to the sex organs.

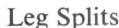
Leg Splits

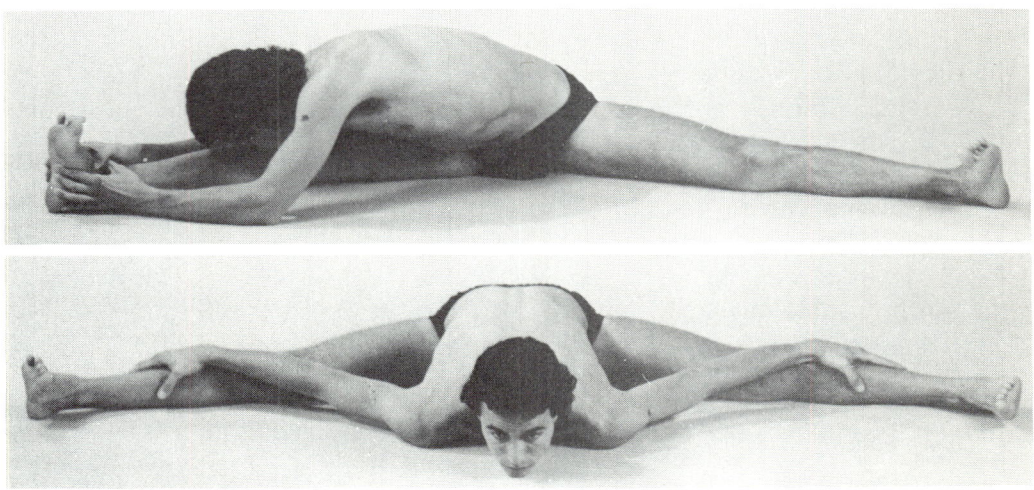

Mahamudra #1 (The Great Yogic Seal)

Extend the right leg as you sit on the ground. Tuck the left heel into the crotch, and hold the right big toe with both hands. The spine is straight, with the chin tucked into the chest. Inhale deeply, and hold the breath for a count of ten. Then exhale

Mahamudra #1

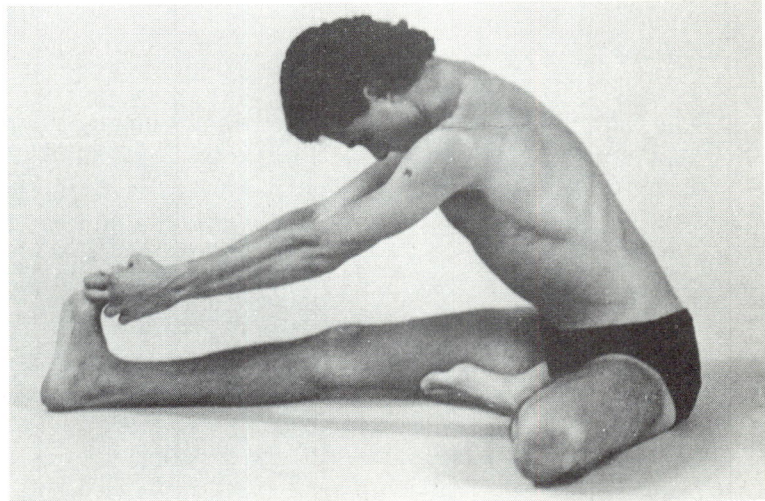

all the way out. Repeat a dozen times or more on each side. Relax after this for a couple of minutes.

Benefits: Strengthens the spine, dramatically increases the flow of energy throughout the entire nervous system, enhances immunity, improves digestion and assimilation, improves skin tone, improves overall vitality.

Mahamudra #2

Extend the right leg as you sit on the ground. Tuck the left heel into the crotch, and hold the right big toe with both hands. The spine is bent forward over the right leg, with the head resting on the knee. Inhale deeply, and hold the breath for a count of ten. Then exhale all the way out. Repeat a dozen times or more on each side. Relax after this for a couple of minutes.

Benefits: Stretches the spine, dramatically increases the flow of energy throughout the entire nervous system, enhances immunity, improves digestion and assimilation, improves skin tone, improves overall vitality.

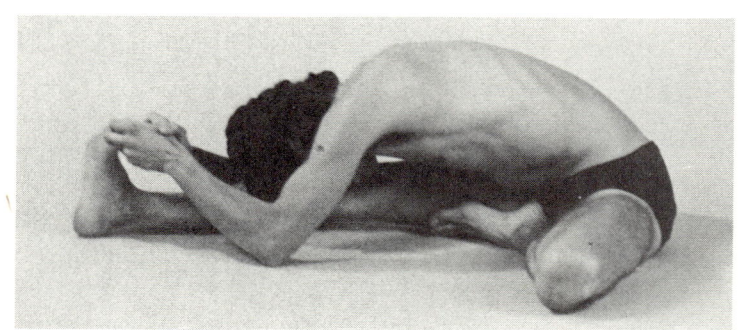

Mahamudra #2

Mahamudra #3

Sit with both legs outstretched together, with your hands grasping the big toes of both feet. Looking up, with the spine straight and stretched up as high as possible, take a deep breath. Then exhale, stretching down over your legs, bringing your head to your knees. Hold the position for a count of five, and then inhale up again. Repeat twenty times.

Benefits: Stretches out the back of the legs, opens up the lower spine, enhances circulation of energy throughout the entire nervous system, purifies the body, increases circulation to the head.

Note: This posture should be avoided by individuals who are chronically constipated.

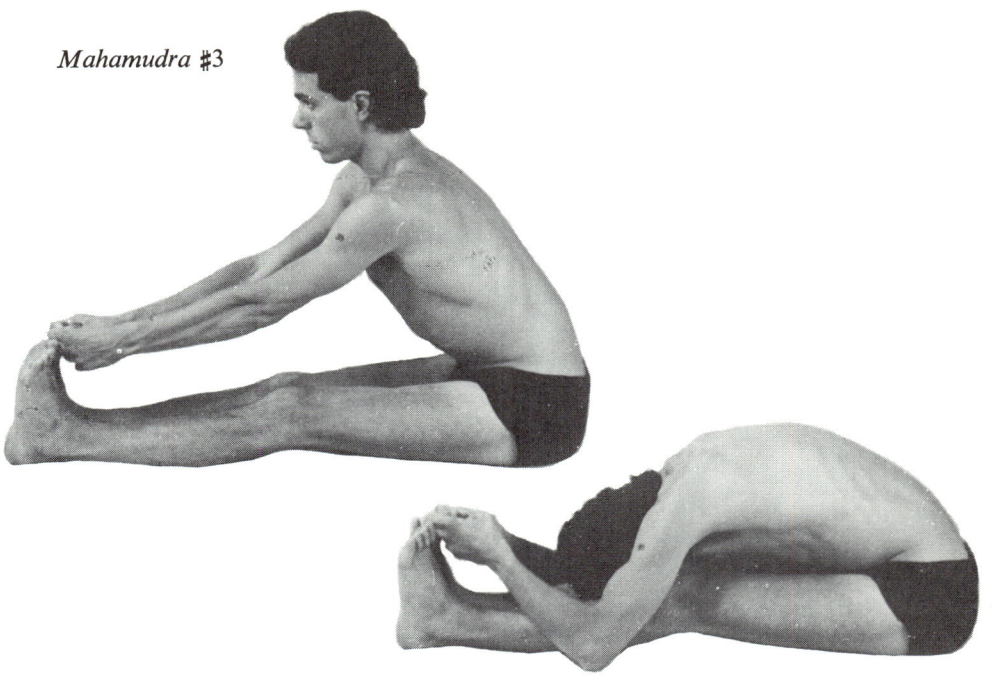

Mahamudra #3

Abdominal Tensor Pose

Sit with the legs together and the trunk upright. Lean back at a 60 degree angle, and raise the legs to a 45 degree angle. The arms are extended on either side of the legs, parallel to the floor. Breathe deeply in this position for a minute.

Benefits: Strengthens the legs, hips, buttocks, abdomen, and back.

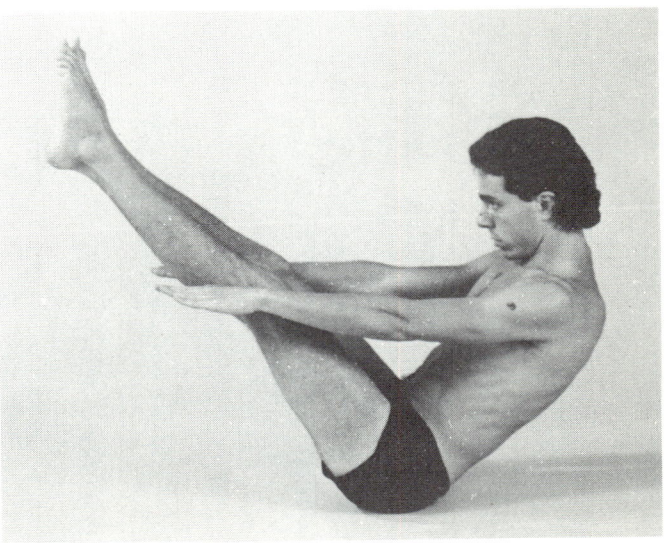

Abdominal Tensor Pose

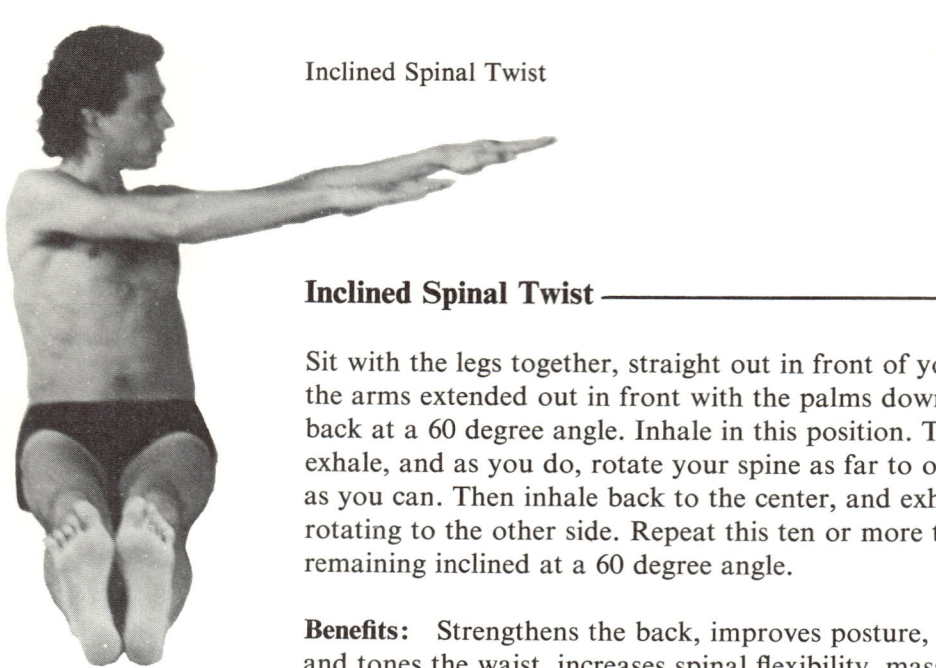

Inclined Spinal Twist

Inclined Spinal Twist

Sit with the legs together, straight out in front of you. With the arms extended out in front with the palms down, lean back at a 60 degree angle. Inhale in this position. Then exhale, and as you do, rotate your spine as far to one side as you can. Then inhale back to the center, and exhale, rotating to the other side. Repeat this ten or more times, remaining inclined at a 60 degree angle.

Benefits: Strengthens the back, improves posture, trims and tones the waist, increases spinal flexibility, massages internal organs.

Spinal Twist

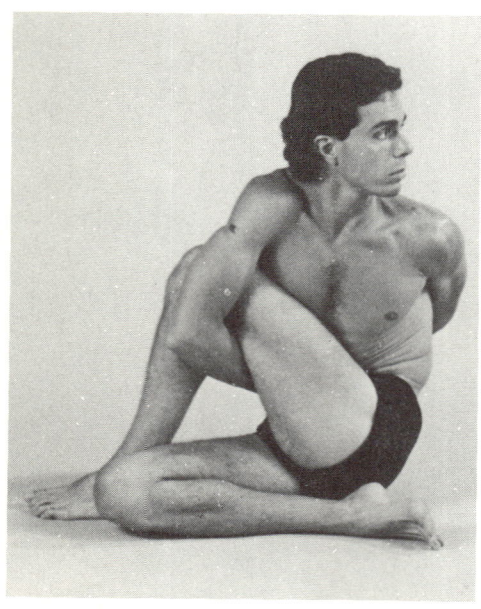

Spinal Twist

Sitting on the ground, stretch your legs out in front of you. Bend your right leg from the knee with the sole of the right foot close to the anus. Bend the left leg while you raise your knee, and keep the left foot flat on the floor to the right side of the right knee.

Stretch the right hand forward and stretch it over the raised knee of the left leg, and grab the big toe of the left foot with your right hand. Stretch your left arm behind you, and grab onto the right hand. Twist your trunk to the left, looking over your left shoulder. In this position, breathe long and deep for a minute or more. Then switch and do the same with the other side.

Benefits: Increases spinal flexibility, improves circulation to the abdominal organs, enhances intestinal activity, improves digestion.

Fish Pose

Sitting upright on the ground, tuck the outer edge of your left foot into the crease of your right hip and inner thigh. Pull your right foot up over your left leg, tucking the outer edge of the right foot into the crease of your left hip and inner thigh. Lean back, arching your spine up toward the sky, resting on the top of your head. Hold onto your feet, and breathe long and deep for a minute or more.

Alternatively, stretch back as before, with the arms stretched back behind your head, holding the opposite elbows with your hands. Breathe long and deep for a minute or more.

Benefits: Increases spinal flexibility, opens up the ribs, opens the lungs, strengthens the neck, increases circulation to the head, enhances the flow of energy throughout the entire nervous system.

Fish Pose

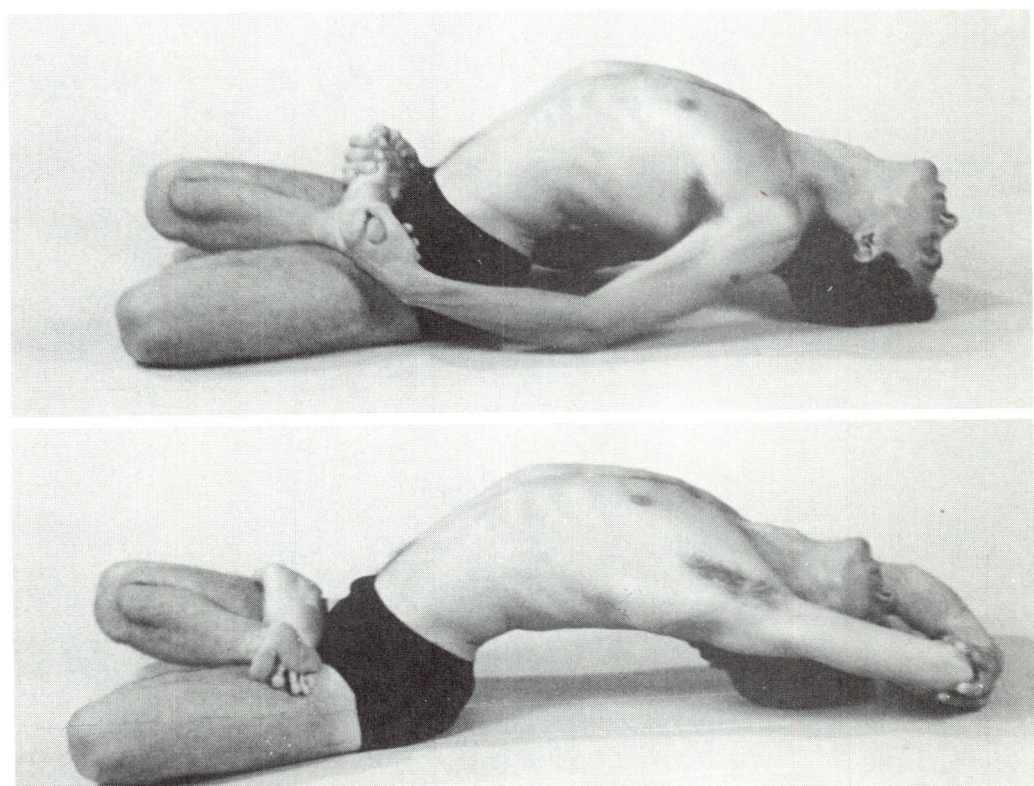

Grasshopper Pose

Lie on the floor on your front, with your arms by your sides with the palms up. Inhale, and raise one leg up behind you, keeping the leg straight. Exhale, and bring it down. Repeat with each leg, inhaling up and exhaling down, twenty times on each side.

Benefits: Strengthens the lower back, improves circulation to the sex organs, digestive organs, and kidneys, and tones the legs.

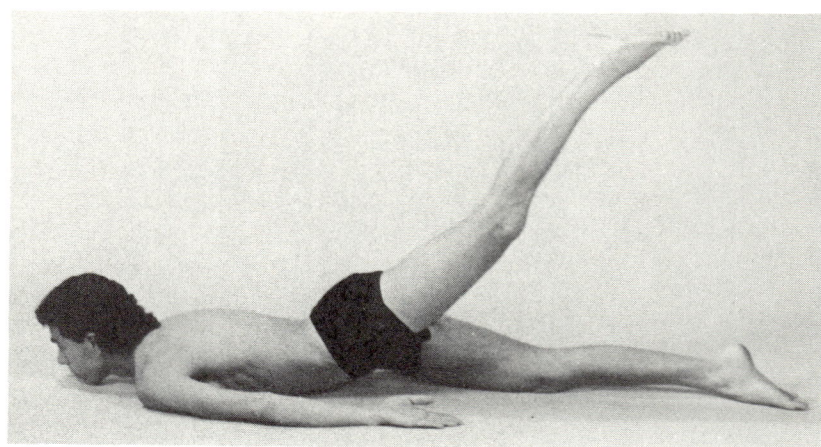

Grasshopper Pose

Locust Pose

Lying flat on your abdomen, make fists with your hands and place them under you, inside the hips and slightly above the pubic bone. Keep your chin on the ground, while you raise your legs behind you, thighs off the ground. In this position breathe

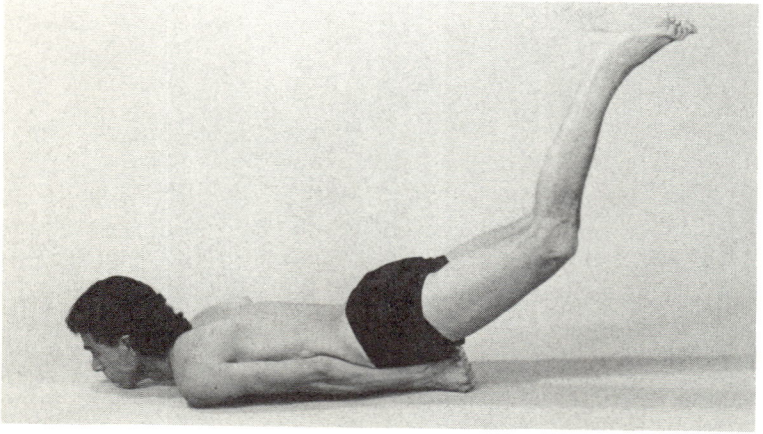

Locust Pose

long and deep for a few seconds, then relax. Build up to being able to do this for a minute.

Benefits: Increases circulation to the pelvis and abdomen, strengthens the lower back and backs of the legs, increases stamina.

Boat Pose

Lie flat on your abdomen with your legs out straight behind you, and your arms out straight in front of you. Raise your legs and chest up, making a boat shape with your body. In this position, breathe long and deep. Try to hold the position for a minute.

Benefits: Increases circulation to the pelvis and abdomen, strengthens the back, shoulders, and chest, tones the backs of the legs.

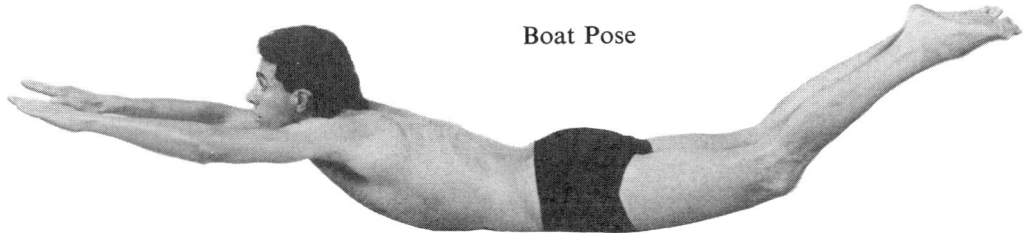

Boat Pose

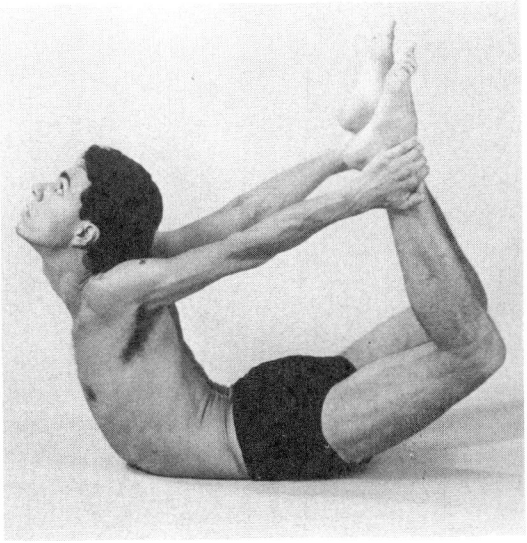

Bow Pose

Bow Pose

Lie on your abdomen, grab hold of your ankles with your hands keeping the arms straight. Raise your head as high as you can and at the same time push the ankles up and back, away from you. Pull yourself up high, so that only a small portion of your midsection remains on the ground. In this position, breathe long and deep for a minute or more.

Benefits: Improves circulation to the pelvis, enhances intestinal activity, improves digestion, strengthens the lower back, stretches the abdomen, opens the lungs and throat.

Cobra Pose

Lie on your abdomen. Place the hands palms down under the shoulders. Raise your head up, looking up and back. Push up with the arms, keeping the thighs on the ground. Your spine will arch as you push up. Stretch up as far as you can, and hold the pose, breathing long and slow. Hold for a minute or more.

Benefits: Increases spinal flexibility, improves posture, enhances digestion, increases intestinal activity, improves circulation to the pelvis, opens the chest and lungs, opens the throat, stretches the neck.

Cobra Pose

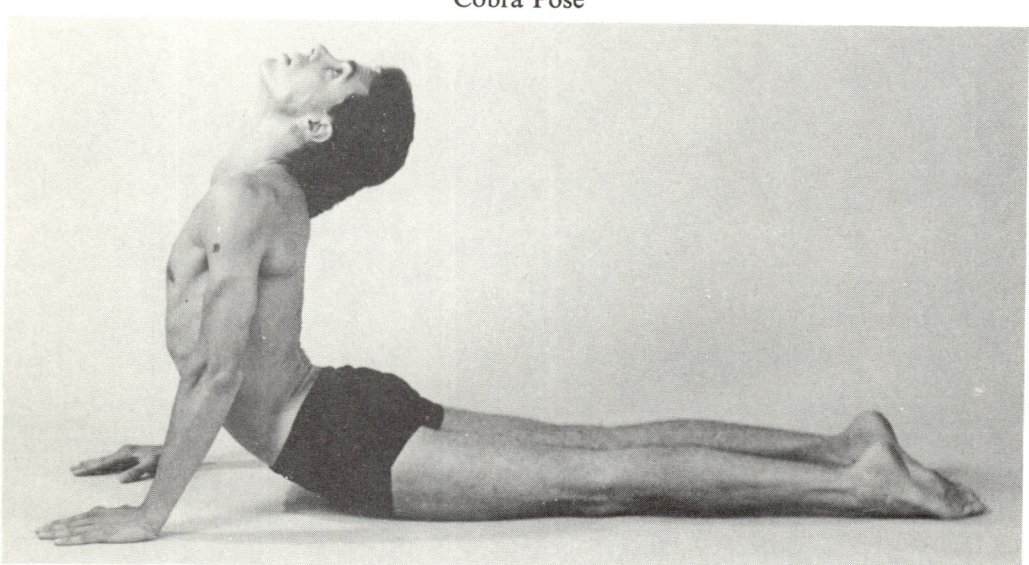

Peacock Pose

With your legs together and your body straight, place the palms down on the ground, with the wrists turned outward with the fingertips pointing toward your feet, and the elbows close to each other. Lean your abdomen on your elbows, and raise your legs off the ground so that your body is parallel to the ground. Breathe normally in this position for up to a minute.

Benefits: Strengthens the back, stimulates the abdominal organs, increases strength and stamina.

Peacock Pose

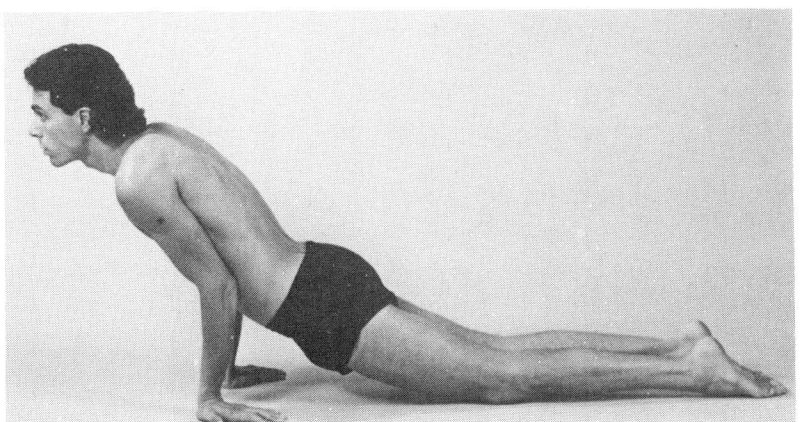

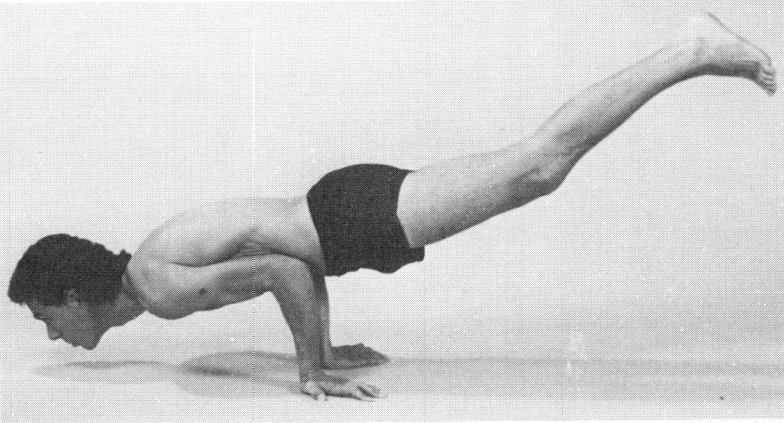

Bridge Pose

Lie on your back with your legs together, bent at the knees, with the feet flat on the ground. Push your hips up toward the sky, supporting your lower back with your hands. Breathe long and deep for a minute or more.

Bridge Pose

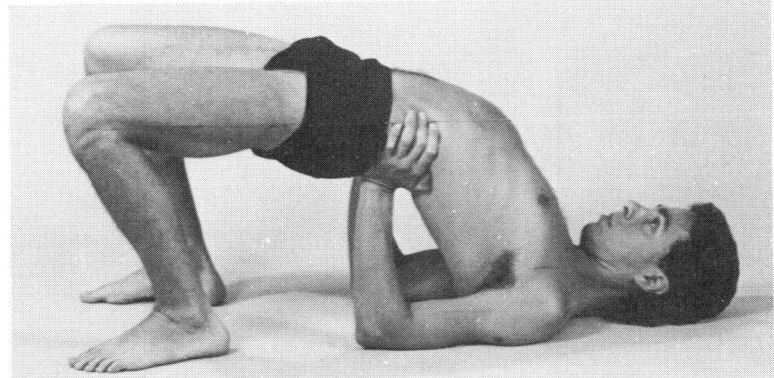

Benefits: Reverses prolapsis, increases spinal flexibility, enhances circulation to the head, increases intestinal activity, strengthens the thighs.

Camel Pose

Stand on the knees, with the insteps of the feet flat on the floor. The knees are about ten inches apart. Lean back, grabbing the heels with your hands. Let your head drop back and push your hips as far forward as possible. In this position, breathe long and deep, for a minute or more.

Benefits: Increases spinal flexibility, opens the lungs and throat, stretches the abdomen, opens the rib cage, loosens the hips, stretches the thighs.

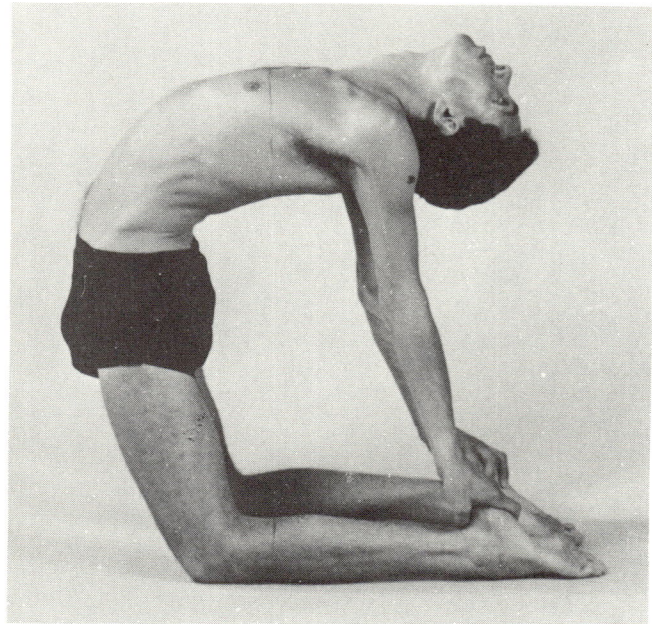

Camel Pose

Inclined Pose

Sit with the legs out straight in front of you, leaning back on the palms of the hands. The palms are pointed straight back, and the arms are straight. Raise the hips so that the entire body is straight, like a plank. In this position, breathe long and deep for a minute or more.

Benefits: Strengthens the back, shoulders, arms, buttocks, and wrists.

Inclined Pose

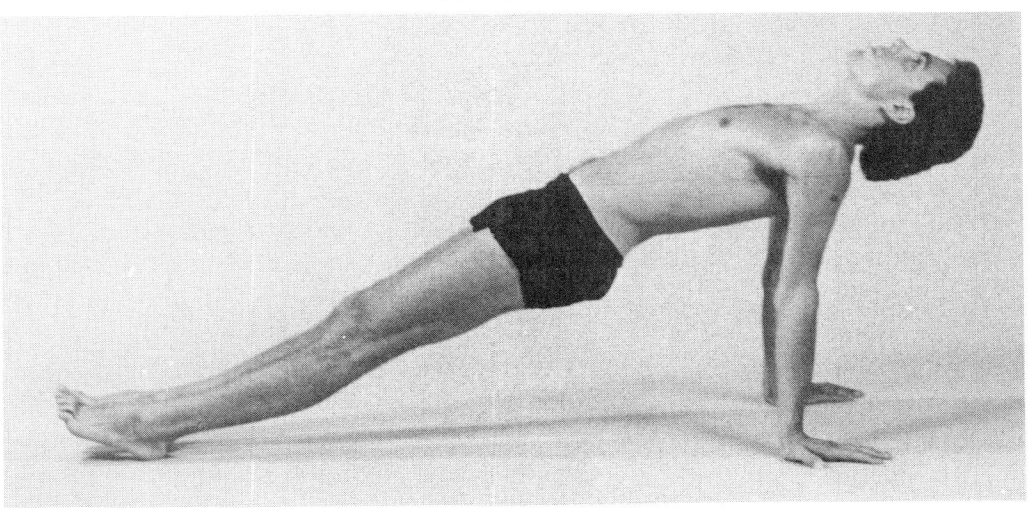

Wheel Pose

Lie on your back with the knees together and the feet flat on the ground tucked up close to the buttocks. Bend your arms back, with the palms of the hands underneath the shoulders, with the fingers pointing toward your feet. Push your hips up, and at the same time push your arms, so that you rest on the top of your head. From there, push yourself up, so that the hips are pressed up toward the sky, and the arms are fully extended. In this position, take ten long, deep breaths.

Wheel Pose

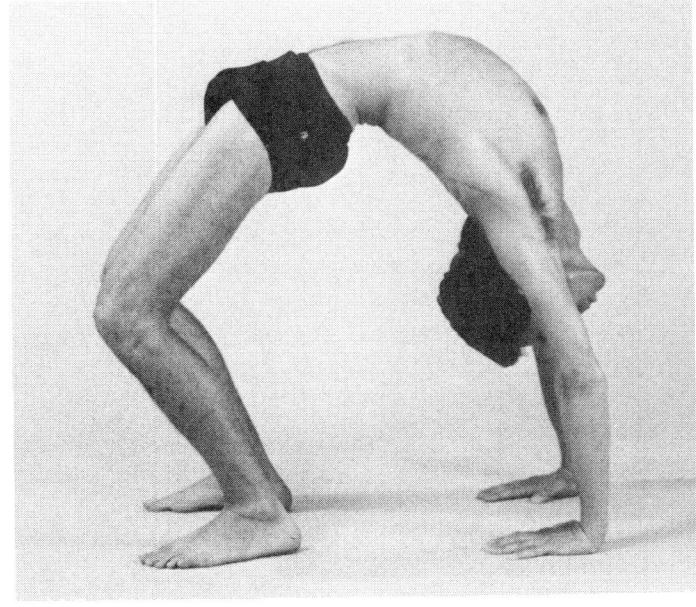

Benefits: Increases spinal flexibility, strengthens the arms and shoulders, opens the chest and lungs, opens the throat, increases circulation to the head.

Plow Pose

Lie on your back with your arms by the sides. With your legs together, extend the legs up and over your head, bringing your feet to the floor behind your head. Stretch back as far as you can. Then, extend your arms behind you, with the hands pointing toward your feet. In this position, breathe normally, stretching a little more with each breath. Stay in this position for a couple of minutes or more.

Benefits: Increases spinal flexibility and flexibility of the backs of the legs, reverses prolapsis, increases circulation to the head.

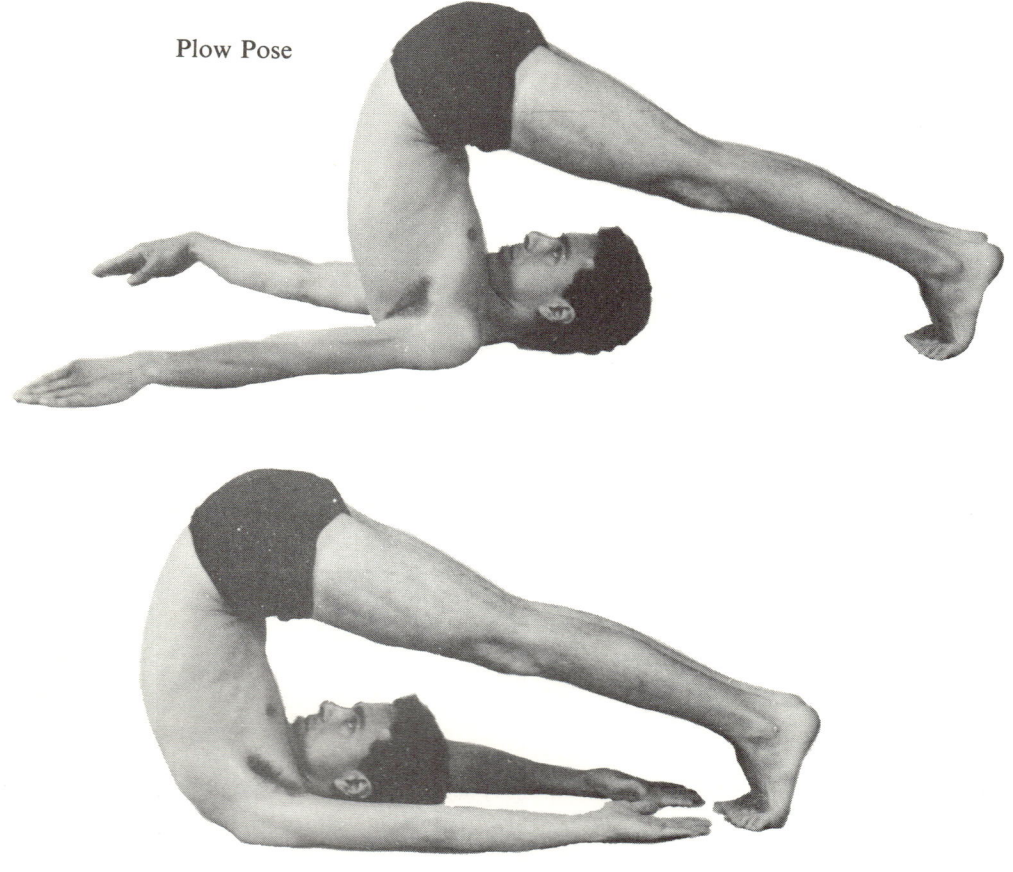

Plow Pose

Reverse Seal

Lie on your back with the legs straight. Raise your legs, as though to move into plow pose. Supporting your hips with your hands, straighten the legs upright.

Reverse Seal

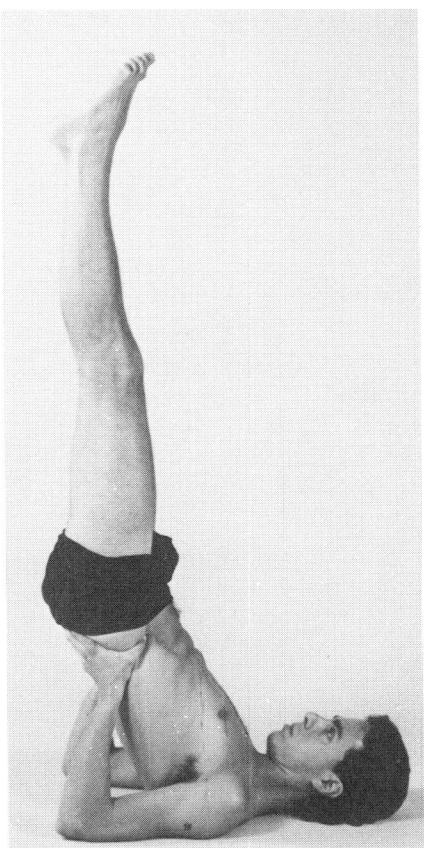

Take a long deep breath and hold for a count of ten. Repeat ten times, then come down.

Benefits: Increases the flow of life energy throughout the entire nervous system, increases the flow of spinal fluid to the brain, improves circulation to the head, reverses prolapsis.

Shoulder Stand

Lie on your back with the legs straight. Raise your legs up and back, as though to go into plow pose. Supporting your mid back with your hands, straighten your entire body so that you are perfectly upright, with the chin tucked into the chest. In this position, breathe normally for a minute or more.

Shoulder Stand

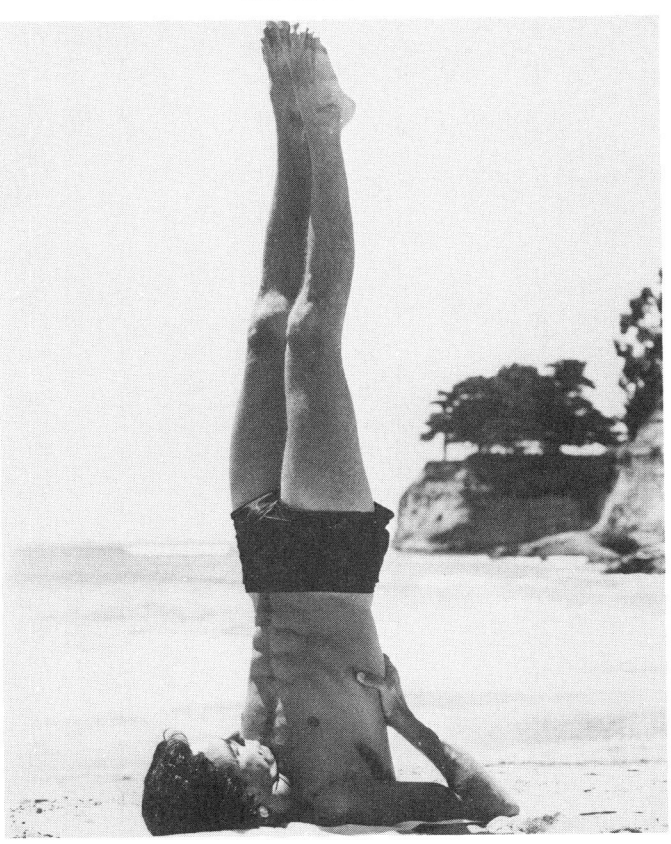

Benefits: Increases the flow of life energy throughout the entire nervous system, increases the flow of spinal fluid to the brain, improves circulation to the head, reverses prolapsis, stimulates the thyroid.

Corpse Pose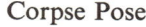

Lie on your back with your legs outstretched, with the feet about eight inches apart. The arms are near the sides, with the palms up. In this position, breathe normally, and as you do, begin to relax all the muscles in your body. With every breath, let go of tension, allowing yourself to go into a deep, deep relaxation. Use Corpse pose to relax after performing all other postures. Allow yourself to rest in this position for at least five minutes; longer is preferred.

Benefits: Allows life energy to flow smoothly throughout the entire body, and enables you to shed stress.

Corpse Pose

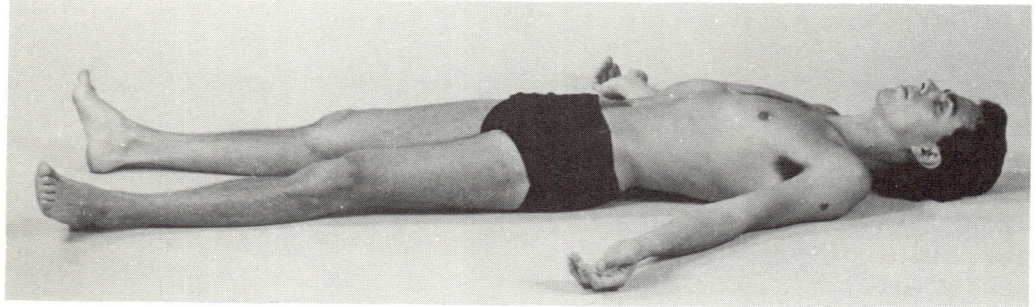

INGREDIENTS of NATURAL LIVING

Nature's Three Great Healers:
Sunshine, Fresh Air, and Pure Water

Sunshine

For as long as human history can recount, the sun has been an object of great reverence and wonder. Nothing else in the visible Universe has commanded such attention, and for good reason. The sun provides heat and light for our small planet, contributing to an atmosphere which supports life, while brilliantly illuminating our days. Intense and durable, the sun allows plants and animals to grow, and makes life possible for us.

Yogis have always emphasized the importance of sunlight to health. Daily exposure is life sustaining, and provides us with many nutrients essential to dynamic living. Modern science knows this to be true, and that exposure to sunlight triggers the body's production of vitamin D, which is important to the proper formation of bones and teeth, healthy hair, and skin. Vitamin D is needed for the utilization of calcium and phosphorous. An inadequate intake of vitamin D can lead to rickets and great loss of energy. For this reason, people who live in cool or cold climates often need to take a vitamin D supplement during the winter months. At that time there is less sunshine, and more time is spent inside.

Sunshine is more than just a source of vitamin D. Sunshine provides basic life energy. When people get enough sunshine, their energy often increases, making them more robust and alive. This is assuming, of course, that other factors in their lives are also life supporting. We have all known people who, having journeyed to Jamaica, Hawaii, or the Caribbean return looking healthy, and feeling energetic. Naturally, the relaxation of vacation time has tremendous prophylactic effects, but it is exposure to the sun that gives tropical visitors the look and feel of health.

Yogis have long claimed that the sun acts upon the endocrine system, balancing the various glands, and enhancing internal harmony. A great deal of research has substantiated this claim. In his book *Health and Light*, Dr. John Ott, a scientific pioneer, goes into great detail to show that full-spectrum light, as provided by the sun, is absolutely essential to total health. Lack of such light, he shows, can lead to a variety of deficiencies and ailments. These studies have led to the successful treatment of some ailments with the use of light. Now an increasing number of health researchers are examining the role that full-spectrum light plays in health.

It is essential to get outside in broad daylight and absorb precious sunshine through the skin and eyes. There are small sites in the eyes, known as retino-receptors, which trigger the function of the entire glandular system. Exposure to full-spectrum sunlight activates balanced glandular activity. Exposure to partial-spectrum light, such as fluorescent tube lighting, stimulates imbalanced glandular activity. When fresh, unfiltered sunlight is taken into the eyes, a series of reactions occurs chemically and in the nervous system. The effect is like a tune-up, causing the glandular system to function more smoothly and harmoniously. This is necessary for internal biochemical balance. It ensures that the thousands of hormones and compounds that we manufacture will occur properly, in the correct amounts.

One of the first recommendations of Yogatherapy is to receive adequate sunlight. Go outside and be active. Walk in the sunshine and drink it through your skin and eyes. This does not mean that you should look directly into the sun. Simply being outside in the sun allows the eyes to absorb full-spectrum light from the sun. Instead of taking a coffee break, take a sun break. Get at least fifteen minutes of sunlight a day, but preferably more. Of course, if you have very sensitive skin or an unusual skin disorder, be judicious and do not expose yourself to too much sun too quickly.

Many natural health care practitioners including myself are of the point of view that it is not the sun which causes skin cancer or spots on the skin. These conditions arise when there is toxicity or chemical imbalance, often related to the liver or intestines. When there is toxicity in the body, exposure to sunlight will bring these toxins to the skin. In this case, the problem is not the sun, but internal pollution, usually caused by inadequate elimination of waste. In case of chemical imbalances, exposure to sunlight may exacerbate the problem. The sun, however, is not the primary cause of the disorder. The problem is a pre-existing condition of imbalance. The solution is not to avoid sunlight, but to correct the imbalance. In the case of toxicity, the problem is internal pollution, and the solution is to cleanse the body of impurities with a safe and effective program. A cleansing diet and treatments for the liver and intestines are given in this book.

The sun is ours to savor and enjoy. Make it a point to get sunshine every day, and feel strength and vitality flowing through you as you do.

Fresh Air

It is known that people can live for extended periods of time without food. One can go without water or sleep for several days, and without companionship for prolonged periods of time. But if you go without air for more than just a few minutes, you will lapse into a coma and die. Thus air is the most essential element taken into the body. Night or day, twenty-four hours daily, for all our lives, we must have air. We must breathe air, and our skin must have contact with air. It is vital for life.

Through both the respiratory system and the skin, air is taken into the body. Oxygen from air does many things. It provides for whole, healthy blood, it nourishes, strengthens, and builds healthy tissue, it stimulates the brain, and enhances energy production. When the body performs hard work, oxygen from breathing contributes to strength and endurance. And when we take a deep, sweeping sigh, that breath is relaxing.

We need air constantly. The air should be fresh, wholesome, and clean, free from all pollution and debris. Unfortunately, however, humanity has carried its excessive indulgences to the point that the air in our environment is polluted with toxic wastes from cars and industrial facilities. This unfortunate result of industry can seriously compromise human and animal health. After all, no matter where we are we must breathe. And no matter what the air is like, we must breathe it. We invariably inhale the pollutants and acrid waste products which litter the air wherever we are.

Fortunately there are still places where the air is clean and fresh, where a deep breath of air is rich and satisfying. Rural areas, the mountains, and the deserts are usually clean and fresh. This is also true at the seashore in some places. It is helpful to get to those areas, if you do not live there, and to breathe deeply. There are marvelous national forests and reserves where wildlife abounds, and where there is still clean air. Vacation time is well spent there, and the air helps to purify and refresh the body/mind.

In some urban areas the air is so polluted that simply breathing the air is equivalent to smoking a pack of cigarettes daily. On top of that, there are people who smoke. Each person pays the price for the headstrong ambition on the part of industry to "get ahead" without paying heed to our precious and limited natural resources, one of which is fresh air.

Yogatherapy recognizes the need for fresh air, and recognizes the value of powerful breathing exercises to cleanse and invigorate the entire system. Go out as often as possible and get fresh air. Be active outdoors, and get away to places which are unpolluted. Make it a point to engage in healthy recreational activities in a natural setting, and breathe deeply. More specific information will be given about dynamic breathing exercises later on. Air is one of Nature's greatest healers—use it for life.

Pure Water

Approximately 70% of our total body weight is water. Two thirds of the surface of the earth is covered with water as well. Water is very important. It provides us with the fluid needed for healthy tissue and blood in our bodies, it allows living things to grow, keeps land from eroding and blowing away, and provides navigable territory to get from one place to another by boat or ship.

Without water we could not live. We would be dust, and the earth would be parched, dry, and uninhabitable. We are fortunate that there is enough water to meet our needs. Yogis have traditionally used water for the restoration and maintenance of health. This is accomplished by both the internal and external uses of water. Drinking and bathing are very important in Yogatherapy, for several reasons.

The body is constantly replenishing itself. New cells are being made, and old cells are being eliminated. Within a seven year period almost every cell in the body is replaced by a new one. All of the functions of growth, renewal and elimination require an ample supply of water. Water is a major constituent of cells, and is the greatest part of the fluids that carry nutrients to make new cells. It is also the primary medium by which dead cells are transported through the body and eliminated. For almost every bodily function, water is required. This water must be kept whole, fresh and clean. Otherwise toxicity can build up, and the body will become polluted. It is just like a stream into which pollutants are poured. If there is not enough fresh water, the water system will finally break down and become virtually useless.

Our body water must be replenished daily. It is necessary to consume an adequate amount of water every day to maintain internal cleanliness, and to replenish depleted water stores. We are constantly giving off water from our bodies. This occurs in four ways. The first is expiration. With every exhalation, some water is lost. If you will breathe onto a piece of glass you will see that this is so. On the glass will accumulate tiny beads of moisture from the breath. More moisture is lost from the body via expiration than by any other means. Secondly there is urination. As fluid passes through the body, it travels through the kidneys and bladder, and is eliminated as urine. Thirdly there is perspiration, by which water is eliminated through the pores of the skin. A healthy body is always perspiring. This is not to say that a healthy person is constantly dripping with sweat, but the body will steadily give off a moderate amount of moisture. This helps to maintain an even body temperature, and keeps the pores of the skin open and well irrigated. Lastly there is defecation, by which water is eliminated through the bowels. This is the least of the ways by which water is eliminated, but is important nonetheless. Many sufferers of chronic constipation have found relief by drinking an ample amount of water daily.

For the purposes of Yogatherapy, it is recommended that you drink approximately six to eight glasses of water daily. Upon rising, drink about a pint of water, preferably warm, with half of a freshly squeezed lemon or lime in it. During the course of the day, try to consume at least six more glasses of water. There are some tips, though. Do not drink heavily before, during, or directly after a meal. Heavy fluid consumption at mealtime can dilute the gastric juices required to digest food, and diminish the concentration of digestive enzymes. Generally it is best to limit yourself to one glass of fluid with a meal.

There are many herbal teas that enhance digestion, and they may be substituted for water with a meal. Herbs will be discussed further on in more detail.

Bathing is also important in Yogatherapy. It is healthful to bathe daily, by taking a shower, a bath, or a swim in clean, fresh, unpolluted waters. When bathing it is advisable to use a loofa sponge, obtainable at most natural food stores, and scrub your entire face and body with that. This will improve circulation, scrub off dead cells from the pores, and massage vital oils back into the skin. With a loofa no soap is needed, though it can be used if desired.

Swimming in a lake, stream, or the ocean is healthful and invigorating for reasons other than cleanliness. Bodies of water such as lakes and oceans have a strong negative ionic charge, which is soothing and energizing to the body. The negative ionic charge is prevalent in the atmosphere near such waters. This is why a person can become invigorated by simply walking along the seashore. There the negative ionic charge is particularly strong, and it quickly stimulates the body. Yogis often bathe in natural bodies of water because of that effect. Swimming and bathing in natural waters is highly recommended, and swimming provides one of nature's most perfect forms of exercise.

There is some controversy among natural health enthusiasts as to whether spring water or pure, distilled water should be drunk. In my opinion, spring water is ideal for consumption. In all the areas of the world where people live to be very old while still healthy, spring water is drunk exclusively. However, if you are in an area where the tap water is impure, and there is no source of spring water, then it is fine to drink distilled water instead.

Water is basic, simple, and essential to life. Drink it, bathe in it, swim in it, and use it. But be conservative, never wasteful. Like all of our precious resources, water is limited and must be protected, lest we spoil it all.

The Benefits of Walking

The most simple and natural of all forms of exercise is walking. Walking is fundamental to Yogatherapy, and is highly beneficial to total health.

Walking strengthens the legs, improves circulation, maintains posture, improves internal organ tone, promotes regularity, and enables the body to produce more energy. Unfortunately, our modern world is more geared toward the automobile and its use than to the practice of walking. However, you can work around this. Whenever it is feasible, you can try walking someplace instead of taking a car. If that means taking twenty or thirty extra minutes to get someplace, make time for that. When you arrive at your destination, you'll feel better for it.

Prior to the development of mechanical means of travel, people walked a great deal, often many miles every day. Times have changed, though, and nowadays people are busy earning a living, and usually have little time to walk. Nonetheless, you can manage to walk two miles a day, either in the morning or evening. To walk that distance takes less than half an hour, an amount of time that almost everybody can set aside. If possible, walk to work instead of taking transportation. When you need to pick up just a few items from the store, walk there. If you do drive to the store, park far from the door, and let everyone else compete for the front row spaces. Whenever possible, get in a little walking.

When walking, try to maintain a brisk pace. This is of more value than maintaining a slow gait, as it stimulates the cardiovascular system. Walking, like Yoga, is wonderful because it can be done at any time, and requires no special apparatus. When you have a free day, instead of plunking down on the living room couch, take a walk. A long walk can be interesting, and provides healthy and cost-free family fun. Whenever time and weather permit, make walking part of your daily health plan.

Sleep

In the Yogic description of the Creation, the Universe goes forth and spreads itself endlessly in all directions. There comes a time, however, when the Universe is recalled, when it returns to the great silence. At that moment there is just darkness and peace. The time of darkness and formlessness is called *Pralaya*. After a while, the Universe springs forth again.

For people, sleep is much like pralaya. It is a time to return to silence, to stillness, to a deep and profound darkness, in which there is rest for the body, the mind, and the soul. The body needs sleep for regeneration and repair. The mind needs sleep to shut down completely, so that it can function fresh again the next day. For the soul, the power of silence enables spiritual energies to flow more freely. Sleep speeds the healing process, and refreshes the entire person. It is an opportunity to recharge and gather new forces.

One's need for sleep is proportionate to the other factors in one's life. However, one thing can be said in general, and that is that all of us must have some profoundly deep rest, as obtained in sleep, or we will become run-down. Unfortunately, even some people who sleep long hours do not get the rest they need. This is where Yogatherapy is of inestimable value. Through diet, exercise, and meditation, one can achieve deeply satisfying, nourishing sleep. Surprisingly, you may find that you actually require less sleep time as a result. I have seen this happen to many people. It is not unusual for someone who eats well, exercises, and meditates to require even one or two fewer hours sleep per night. Besides enabling one to sleep less and feel rested, Yogatherapy increases energy and clarity of mind. Thus you not only need to sleep less, but are more dynamic during waking hours.

There are a few recommendations which can make sleep more enriching for you. It is ideal to sleep on your back, in "corpse pose," with legs straight out, the arms near the sides with the palms up. In this position, take a few deep breaths and relax gradually. You will pass into a deep sleep. If, however, you sleep lightly or are frequently beset by bad dreams, sleep on your right side. By sleeping on the right side you will automatically breathe predominantly through the left nostril, which has a calming effect. This will enable you to sleep more deeply, with less disturbance. If, on the other hand, you usually sleep well but would like more energy upon awakening, then sleep on your left side. In this position the right nostril is blowing, and you will be energized as you sleep.

Sleep on a firm surface, in a well ventilated room. It is unhealthy to sleep in a closed room, as you breathe the same air over and over again. Make sure that there is fresh air in the room by sleeping with a window open.

Allow yourself maximum comfort when you sleep. Sleep either in clothing which is non-restrictive, or better yet, in no clothes at all. Make sure that your covers are adequate so that you do not get chilled at night. Most importantly, though, empty your mind when you go to bed. Sleep is for rejuvenation and refreshment, so don't let yourself be bogged down by thoughts or problems. Sleep deeply, and you will be better equipped to deal with everything else later on.

Hot and Cold Showers

The therapeutic use of different types of baths of varying temperatures comprises the health system of hydrotherapy. In hydrotherapy, baths are used in specific ways for a variety of health problems. This type of treatment is very effective, and has been proven to help remedy many of the most obstinate health disorders known.

One of the simplest prophylactic techniques of hydrotherapy is to take a hot shower followed by a cold one each morning. This simple bathing procedure works wonders for overall health. In the first place, by taking a hot shower followed by a cold one, the circulation in the body is greatly increased, allowing the blood to flush deep into the internal organs, and to the extremities as well.

Secondly, the cold shower following the hot one closes pores, strengthens the nervous system, and strengthens the adrenal glands, thereby enhancing stamina. This showering procedure is effective in building resistance to colds, and body temperature stays warmer in chilly conditions. I have noticed that this simple hydrotherapy practice has enabled me to be warm in conditions which once would have chilled me.

The procedure to follow is this: Get into a shower and make the water as hot as is comfortable. In the hot shower, scrub yourself thoroughly with a brush or loofa sponge. This will clean you and massage your skin. After you have washed, shampooed, or whatever else you need to do, then turn the water to cold. Initially as you start to get accustomed to the cold water, you may wish to make it just cool. That's fine. In time you will be able to turn the water all the way to the coldest setting without any difficulty at all. In fact, it can be very enjoyable.

With the cold water shooting at you, massage your body with your hands as the water runs over your skin. Rub your face, underarms, and all parts of your body, while under the water spray. Put your back up against the cold water and let it flow against your lower back and kidney area. This stimulates the adrenal glands, and helps to firm sagging buttocks as well. A thorough cold shower will take about two minutes. When you are done you will feel great.

The hot and cold shower treatment is particularly efficacious in the morning before Yoga practice, as it wakes you up completely. If the water pressure in your shower is adjustable, increase the force of the flow, as this will enhance the benefits of the entire procedure. The hot and cold shower will add energy and vitality to your day.

Regularity in Schedule and Habits

From the Yogatherapy point of view, regularity in schedule and habits is one of the keys to a healthy life. We breathe in rhythm, our hearts beat in rhythm, and our brain waves pulsate in rhythm. To establish a rhythm of schedule and habits is consonant with the natural needs and operation of the body and mind.

Each person is an exquisitely intricate bioenergetic complex, whose multi-functional systems have the capacity for a broad spectrum of tasks. Just as an automobile will last long and run well if it is driven carefully, washed regularly, and tuned and repaired at the appropriate times, so does the human bioenergetic system respond well to regular care. A living schedule is most enjoyable when it meets ones optimal functional needs. It is not necessary to be rigid and compulsive about a living schedule, but it is advantageous to develop a natural rhythm by which to live healthfully. It is a known fact that hectic, stressful, fast-paced living is not conducive to either health or longevity. A life of irregular eating, off-beat sleep habits, fluctuating rising and retiring times, tidal mood changes, and erratic mental and emotional states will not be a long or comfortable life at all.

The human bioenergy system is at its most efficient and balanced functional level when there is a consistent and rhythmic life pattern. This does not necessarily mean a strict schedule, but rather one which easily accommodates the essential factors of daily living. Some of these factors are rising, eating, working, sleeping, Yoga, relaxation, spending time with friends and loved ones, meditation, and having fun. If you can construct your day such that you can accommodate these according to order of priority and practical considerations, you will have an operational base from which to work.

Initially, establishing a balanced schedule for yourself may be both new and difficult. But after a while, you will find that such a rhythm is not restrictive, but allows for enormous personal freedom.

NUTRITION

Diet and Yogatherapy

A healthy diet is a cornerstone of Yogatherapy. The food you eat plays a major role in maintaining a strong, healthy body. This is because food is more than just fuel for energy. It provides the essential building blocks of tissues, bones, and blood. Your tissues need protein to remain strong and supple, and your glands and organs need a variety of vitamins, minerals, and trace elements to operate at peak levels. In addition, you require carbohydrates and fats for energy. At all times, billions of enzymes work within the body as catalysts, triggering countless chemical reactions. Body chemistry is so complex that we have yet to understand the processes that occur in the body in just one minute. It is known, however, that proper nutrition is essential for keeping the body running in a healthy state, without disease or failure.

Everything you eat either contributes to or detracts from your total vitality. Vital foods provide nutrients for dynamic energy, while other junk items actually deteriorate the delicate chemical balance needed for health. It is important, therefore, to maintain a diet that will best serve your health. Currently there are so many diets or eating plans, including the omnivorous, carnivorous, vegetarian, fruitarian, sproutarian, vegan, macrobiotic, juicarian, high protein, high carbohydrate, salt free, and other plans. Every week, a new book hits the newsstands, with a brand new plan that will supposedly meet everyone's needs, help everyone to lose weight, and restore energy to those who have lost it. Such claims are erroneous, though, because no single diet plan is appropriate for everyone. This is because everyone is biochemically unique.

The Yogatherapy diet plan is a time tested, wholesome, tasteful, nutritious way of eating, which allows for variations in individual needs. This diet has been used by thousands of people, with beneficial results. The emphasis here is on high quality, nutritionally rich foods, elimination of junk foods from the diet, and observance of sensible eating habits. Let's examine the major components of the Yogatherapy eating plan.

Vital Foods

Vital foods are foods with life, brimming with essential nutrients just as nature grew them, and prepared with a minimum of processing. They provide optimal nourishment without being hazardous to your health, and they retain a perfect balance of life-sustaining elements, along with a generous supply of vital life force. Life force, the intrinsic factor within all living things, is as nourishing as protein, vitamins, and minerals, and every bit as essential to optimal health. Vital foods contain life energy, and when they are eaten they support the life force which courses through every cell of your body. The main groups of vital foods follow:

Fresh Vegetables and Fruits

Fresh vegetables and fruits are brimming with life. They are the best sources of vitamins and minerals. In addition, they are loaded with enzymes, which are the biological catalysts involved in virtually every bodily function. The enzymes from fresh produce enhance digestion and absorption of nutrients, supporting the body's own natural functions. Fresh fruits and vegetables are superior to canned or frozen goods. This is because many enzymes, vitamins and minerals are lost during cooking, especially at high temperatures. Thus canned or frozen foods contain only a fraction of their original nutritional value, and are no longer vital foods.

If you are not used to eating fresh vegetables, then you are in for a treat. A salad, properly built, can be a meal in itself, delicious and satisfying. If you eat at least one large raw vegetable salad daily, you will be supplying your body with a tremendous amount of nutrition. Raw vegetables supply vitamins, minerals, enzymes and fiber. Fiber is important, as it adds bulk to the bowels and helps to keep them clean. Many illnesses originate from inadequate intestinal elimination, and the regular consumption of fresh salads helps to avoid that problem. Leafy green vegetables such as spinach, chard, kale, and beet greens, also contain chlorophyll, which provides the body with extra oxygen at a cellular level, while acting at the same time as an internal disinfectant and antibacterial agent.

Due to variations in individual digestive ability, some people will tolerate a higher percentage of raw foods in their diet than others. Anyone considering major dietary changes should do so slowly, being observant of any discomfort such as indigestion or gas.

If you do cook your vegetables, steam or sauté them lightly instead of boiling or frying them. Avoid using aluminum cookware, as it can raise body aluminum levels to a toxic point. Carefully prepared vegetables will be juicy and flavorful, retaining most of their nutrients.

Fresh fruit makes a wonderful breakfast and is the ideal snack. Fruits also supply vitamins, minerals, enzymes and fiber. They are generally cleansing and provide natural sugars for energy. Most fruits require a lot of sunshine to grow. Thus they are full of vital energy from the sun, the greatest energy source for our planet. When fresh, ripe fruits are eaten, the rich energy they contain stimulates the body's life force, enhancing overall vitality.

Fresh vegetables and fruits contain many of the nutrients essential to the building and maintenance of healthy bodies. Vitamins A, C, E, and the B-complex, plus the minerals, calcium, magnesium, phosphorous, potassium, zinc, and iodine are just a few of these elements. They are obtained from carrots, broccoli, strawberries, bananas, asparagus, and hundreds of other delicious produce items. By including these foods in your diet, you are making an investment in total health. •

Fresh Juices

While whole, fresh vegetables and fruits are important to the diet, their freshly extracted juices are yet another bonus to good health. Fresh juices are unique foods. They are pure, concentrated, liquid nutrition, containing the health-bestowing essence of the foods from which they are derived. Loaded with vitamins, minerals, enzymes, and natural sugars, fresh juices are easy to digest, are absorbed quickly into the body, and provide high quantities of daily nutritional requirements.

Fresh juices can work wonders for your overall energy level. Since they are packed with essential nutrients, they are among the best foods for activating the full power of the body. As the pure, liquid vitality of fresh juices streams through the body, internal chemistry is stimulated to peak performance. Weak digestive organs are rejuvenated when you drink fresh juices, as there is little work required to reap the benefits of these vital, liquid foods. You will find that if you substitute fresh juices for one meal daily, you will feel lighter, stronger and more energetic. Over a period of time you will see how this makes you feel more dynamic and vital.

In order to obtain fresh juices, you need a juicer. These are expensive appliances, but they last a long time and are an investment in good health. Most natural food stores carry several brands of juicers, though I personally recommend the Champion Juicer. The reason that it is so important to drink juices fresh is that bottled or canned products have minimal nutritional value due to the manner in which they are processed or packaged. Bottled and canned juices have been heated, thereby destroying most of the enzymes and vitamins in them. Even if the juices have not been heated, they are so sensitive to the effects of oxidation that they lose a great deal of nutritional value even when stored under refrigeration. Freshly extracted juices are preferred, because they are the only nutritionally viable juices you can drink, containing the maximum nutritional value.

Besides being generally nutritious, juices also have specific nutritive and therapeutic values. A variety of juices are recommended for various health disorders. These recommendations are based on the specific concentrated nutrients found in particular juices, which thus have particular therapeutic activity. In general, fresh vegetable juices are more nutritionally concentrated than fruit juices. However, both vegetable and fruit juices are used in Yogatherapy to balance body chemistry and establish harmony.

Nuts and Seeds

There are few foods which are as concentrated in their vital, life-bestowing power as raw nuts and seeds. Seeds are the very essence of plant life. They contain the entire life code for plants which are often thousands of times their size. In the world of vegetation, nuts and seeds are the unsurpassed champions of sexual potency and fertility. The similarity between them and our own sperm and eggs is apparent. They each provide the fundamental basis for whole, new living beings.

Nuts and seeds provide vitamins, minerals, essential fatty acids, and protein. They are among the most nutritious of all foods, and have been used traditionally in many cultures to restore flagging vitality.

Common nuts and seeds include Brazil nuts, cashews, chestnuts, coconuts, filberts, flaxseeds, hickory nuts, macadamia nuts, pecans, pistachios, almonds, sesame seeds, and walnuts. They are best eaten raw, for three reasons. First of all, roasting them kills the enzymes within them. Secondly, the same heating process destroys many of their vitamins. Thirdly, the oils in the nuts and seeds become difficult to digest when they are heated. When eaten raw, these small, power-packed foods are nutritional gems.

Nuts and seeds offer protein, which is important for the building of all tissue, for defending the body against disease, and for repairing the body, whenever the need arises. Men need protein for the continuous production of sperm, which is protein-rich, while women need protein to maintain a healthy menstrual cycle.

Essential fatty acids, found in nuts and seeds, are beneficial to overall health. They are required in many reproductive functions, for a healthy prostate gland and normal menstruation, and are of great value to the adrenal glands. The adrenal glands defend the body against stress and fatigue, and also secrete aldosterone, which helps regulate levels of sodium and potassium in the body. Essential fatty acids found in nuts and seeds also produce prostaglandins, hormone-like substances in the body which are involved in metabolism, reproduction, blood circulation, immunity, and nerve function.

Nuts and seeds can be eaten with meals, or as snacks by themselves or with fruit. Nuts store well, are easily portable, and can make a solid contribution to health and vitality.

Dairy Products and Eggs

Among the most highly revered foods for vitality are milk and milk products, and fresh eggs. Even as far back as a couple of thousand years ago, ancient health texts extolled the virtues of these foods for health and virility. There are many reasons that this is so. Dairy products and eggs are high in complete protein, they contain vitamins and minerals, and they are easy for many people to digest. It should be pointed out, however, that a high percentage of Africans and Asians have difficulty digesting milk products, because those population groups do not typically manufacture the digestive enzyme lactase, which is needed for the digestion of milk. However, Indo-Europeans have no trouble with this, in most cases.

Raw, unpasteurized, nonhomogenized milk is preferable to pasteurized and homogenized milk. While it is true that pasteurization is a process employed to kill pathogenic bacteria in milk, the same process also destroys the friendly bacteria which are found naturally in milk, and whose job it is to destroy unhealthy microbes. Dairies that are certified to produce raw milk and raw milk products must undergo continous and rigorous inspections to ensure absolute cleanliness at all times. As a result, these dairies are more sanitary than those from which pasteurized milk products are obtained. Several independant laboratory reports have shown that certified raw milk products are far lower in harmful bacteria than their pasteurized counterparts.

There is another problem with pasteurization. When milk is heated during that process, the casein (milk protein) changes in composition, and becomes harder to digest, forming a glue-like substance. When cooked further, this same milk protein is made into white carpenter's glue. The casein in raw milk, however, is much easier to digest. In fact, many people who cannot tolerate pasteurized milk have no difficulty with raw milk or milk products.

Homogenization is a process by which the fat globules in milk are broken down into tiny particles, so that the cream remains suspended throughout the milk, rather than rising to the top. However, when the milk fat is broken down in such small particles, it bypasses the digestive process, is absorbed into the bloodstream, and can build up as fatty deposits in the arteries. Thus it is more healthful to consume milk that is not only raw, but has not been homogenized as well.

Cultured milk products, such as yogurt, *kefir*, acidophilus milk, and buttermilk are the best to consume, as they are very easy to digest, and they fortify the population of friendly bacteria found in the digestive tract.

Commercially available eggs, as found in most supermarkets, are from chickens which have been kept in very small cages, and fed antibiotics and hormones to maintain a high level of egg production. Besides the fact that the treatment of commercial laying hens is inhumane, the chemicals fed to the birds are passed on in the eggs. The drugs and hormones in the eggs can cause health problems for consumers. There is, however, an alternative. At natural food stores you can purchase farm-fresh, fertile eggs from free-running chickens.

These eggs are higher in nutrients because the chickens are fed better food. The eggs contain no drugs or hormones, so they pose no health hazard to the consumer. Plus, the chickens are raised in a more humane manner. Eggs offer perfect protein, and can make an outstanding contribution to a healthy nutritional plan.

Whole Grains

Historically speaking, the most widely used staple foods have been whole cereal grains, such as wheat, oats, barley, rice, millet, buckwheat, and corn. These foods make up a major portion of the world's food supply, and for good reason—they are packed with nutrition. Whole grains are powerful foods. They are both the seeds and fruits of tall cereal grasses. Everything needed to grow sturdy, healthy plants can be found in the tiny kernels of grains. Like nuts and seeds, grains are highly concentrated nutrition.

Grains are brimming with life force. They grow in the sunshine and absorb a tremendous amount of solar power, the same solar power that helps us to grow. So when you consume grains, you are absorbing accumulated solar energy, in addition to a variety of nutrients. Every day there are new discoveries being made about the life-giving properties of whole grains. For example, it has recently been discovered that there is a substance in whole wheat known as octacosanol. Octacosanol is a stamina factor, a superconcentrated nutrient which imparts enormous strength and endurance when eaten regularly, and which enhances recovery after exertion. It is only present in the germ, however. When whole wheat is ground into white flour, all the octacosanol is lost. What is left is an inferior food which has lost a full 83% of the nutrients found in the whole grain.

The story is the same with other grains. They are powerful, nutrient-rich foods which can enhance health and vitality. But when they are processed and refined they lose their potency. It is for this reason that whole grains and whole grain products are preferred over their refined counterparts. In natural food stores you will find a large assortment of these products, along with information on how to prepare them. Included in your daily diet, whole grains will make a solid contribution to your nutritional status, and thus to your health.

Meats and Fish

It may seem surprising to find meats and fish listed in a book on Yoga and diet, because the traditional Yogic diet is a strict vegetarian plan. However, it must be recognized that a vegetarian diet is not necessarily suitable for everyone. As stated before, each person is biochemically unique. Some function beautifully on a strict meatless program, while other people must have flesh foods to suit their own metabolic requirements. Since Yogatherapy is based on actual nutritional needs, rather than upon a dogmatic religious or philosophical point of view, meats and fish should be considered for their nutritional value.

The best meats to eat for health are the lighter meats, such as poultry, fish and seafoods. Meat provides good quality protein. However, red meats are best eaten sparingly, if at all, for a couple of reasons. In the first place, red meats are high in both uric and lactic acids. These two products build up in the body, and can create an overly acid condition in the blood. This can put a strain on the liver and the kidneys, creating internal toxicity, fatigue, and irritability. Another factor worthy of consideration is that most red meat comes from animals which have been fed drugs, including amphetamines and steroids. Unfortunately, these drugs remain in the meat and can cause serious problems for consumers. Steroids, which are hormones, are of particular concern. They are used to produce rapid growth and weight gain in animals, to make more money per pound of meat for less expense and effort over a shorter period of time. The results of this sound business logic can be disastrous, however. One commonly used steroid, diethylstilbestrol (DES), causes impotence in males and uterine cancer in women. It's hardly worth it for a good steak. Also, since red meats normally turn gray quickly after cutting under normal conditions, they are routinely coated with odorless and tasteless chemicals (including floor-cleaning agents) to keep them red. These chemicals can be poisonous when consumed. So, unless you can get certified organically grown meats through a natural food store, it is best to steer clear of red meats.

It is gradually becoming easier to obtain poultry which has not been fed chemicals, due to consumer demand. Many natural food stores and supermarkets now carry poultry which has been raised without drugs and hormones. In time, availability of these products will surely increase as consumer awareness grows. Poultry such as chicken and turkey is good protein, and does not have the same high uric and lactic acid content as red meats. Plus, poultry is a lighter meat and is easier to digest.

Fish and seafoods are excellent sources of protein. Except from polluted waters, fish is the cleanest and safest of all flesh foods. It is an excellent source of vitamins and minerals, and is lower in fat than red meats. Fish can be eaten regularly as a protein source in the diet, and there is an endless variety of fish to choose from.

Meats, fish, and seafoods are best eaten fresh. Canned or frozen foods lose nutritional value in processing and storage, and do not retain the flavor of fresh products.

What to Avoid

Just as there are foods and substances which make a healthful contribution to the body/mind, so there are agents which are best left alone. Abstaining from the consumption of various substances, including certain foods, is important to the success of your health program. We will briefly examine some of these health destroyers, and what they do.

SUGARS: White, bleached, refined, crystallized, powdered, brown, or so-called "raw" sugars, plus corn syrup, fructose, and table syrups, are high carbohydrate, no-nutrient junk foods. Sugar can damage the liver, adrenal glands, pancreas, teeth, gums, and vitamin/mineral balance of the body. Consumption of sugar can lead to diabetes, which is one of the most disastrous of all common diseases. As much as 70 percent of the American adult population may have some sort of sugar-related disorder. Virtually all commercial brands of cereal, canned vegetables and fruits contain sugar. Pies, cakes, cookies, candies, ice cream and pastries are loaded with the stuff. It shows up in breads, packaged dinners, and most convenience foods. As an alternative to sugar and sugar-laden foods, try fresh fruit. For an occasional sweetener, use honey, but use it in moderation. The body is not designed to handle large amounts of sugar. Any concentrated sweetener or sweet food should be used in moderation, if at all, as they have a profound impact upon the level of sugar in the blood.

WHITE FLOUR: Stripped, refined, degermed, bleached, unbleached, or "enriched" white flour is simply an overprocessed starch whose sole redeeming value is that it can be made into fluffy baked goods. Most commercial brands of breads and baked goods are made exclusively or primarily with white flour. When white flour is made from whole grains, the greatest percentage of nutrients is stripped away, leaving only the starchy, pulpy endosperm inside.

Instead of eating white flour products, eat whole grain foods. They have more flavor, are more nutritious, and can help to prevent a plethora of health problems. Refined flours are difficult to digest, and often cause constipation, which in turn can create internal toxicity, allergies, and many other health problems. Whole grain products, on the other hand, not only have all the natural vitamins and minerals found in grains, but also contain adequate amounts of fiber, which is essential for keeping the bowels clean and moving.

CAFFEINE PRODUCTS: Coffee, colas, regular teas, and a variety of soft drinks contain caffeine, a powerful drug which acts upon the nervous system. It is damaging to the nerves, liver, kidneys, adrenal glands, and nerves. Caffeine upsets the biochemical balance of the body, and regular use can lead to dependancy. Research has implicated caffeine in fibrocystic disease, a painful swelling of the breasts. Caffeine consumption is also associated with some birth defects. Thus caffeine must be used with caution if at all. A cup of tea a couple of times a week will probably do no harm, but regular consumption of caffeine on a daily basis can be hazardous to your health. Most people use caffeine for a lift, as it stimulates the activity of adenosine, an energy producing compound manufactured in the body. However, if you are eating well and following the Yogatherapy plan for health and vitality, you will not have to rely upon caffeine to start your internal engine each day.

CHOCOLATE: Chocolate is actually an addicting food, which contains theobromine, an alkaloid whose properties are similar to those of caffeine. Theobromine is a diuretic and smooth muscle relaxant, and is also a heart stimulant and vasodilator. Chocolate has a powerful drug-like action upon some people. It should be eaten in great moderation, if eaten at all.

PRESERVATIVES AND CHEMICAL ADDITIVES: Preservatives, colors, flavor enhancers, and artificial sweeteners are all chemically manufactured food additives. These products extend the shelf life of foods while they diminish your own chances of reaching old age. They are known to cause cancer, hyperactivity in children, allergies, impotence, nervous disorders, and other health problems. The reason that these agents are used is purely financial. A well preserved box of cereal, for example, can sit on the grocery store shelf for years, without any significant change in appearance or taste. But this never justifies the potential health risk. You can obtain pure, tasty natural foods which contain absolutely no chemical additives. You have a choice; you do not have to be a victim of big business operated by small minds. If you want health and wish to minimize your risk of disease, stay away from foods which contain chemical additives.

ALCOHOL: Almost every adult has an occasional drink, and many drink regularly. Alcohol is an irritant, as well as a powerful drug. As an irritant, it breaks down healthy tissue, particularly that of the brain and glands. As a drug, alcohol is classified as a sedative-hypnotic. Its initial effects include a mild stimulation and a sense of well-being. Heavier consumption produces less lucidity, leading all the way to blind, staggering drunken stupor. Alcohol has historically been used as a general anesthetic due to its powerful ability to deaden nerves. Its use, in anything other than moderation, will deaden nerves and weaken glands to the point that the body and mind can no longer function at a peak level.

Should you drink at all? The answer must be made on an individual basis. An occasional glass of wine or beer will do no harm to many adults. But anything more than that can erode quality of life. Hard alcohol should certainly be avoided, as it has virtually no life-sustaining properties. Remember, your body/mind will only be as attuned and sensitive as you allow it to be. Either keep away from alcohol entirely, or use it with great care, in moderation.

DRUGS: You don't have to rely on Valium, cocaine, speed, depressants, laxatives, or any of the thousands of over-the-counter, under-the-counter, or around-the-corner drugs currently available. Prescription, nonprescription, and recreational drugs all have one thing in common—they all have side effects. Even aspirin, one of the most widely used over-the-counter drugs in the world, can kill a person. Prescription drugs are yet more lethal. When you are given a prescription, ask to see the PDR, the Physician's Desk Reference. There you will find details concerning the potential hazards of the drug you are being advised to take. If your need is not critical, you may wish to pursue alternatives to drug therapy. Competent holistic health practitioners can help you make choices which may save you from the deleterious and sometimes life-threatening effects of drugs.

As for most recreational drugs, there is little use for them if you have a sense of fulfillment and adequate inner resources. If you don't have those things, then drugs dull your inner dissatisfaction, forestalling the day when you will have to come to terms with yourself and figure out how to make your life work. A clear, well-honed mind is more exciting and satisfying than any drug-induced state.

SMOKING: Smoking causes cancer, birth defects, heart disease, respiratory disorders, allergies, bad breath, and other health problems. Smoking has no nutritive or therapeutic value, is a nuisance to others, can be a fire hazard, and unquestionably reduces life span. Smoking is addictive, and expensive. It is a habit without redemption. Don't smoke.

That covers the major things to avoid. If you take care of your body/mind, you will enjoy a high quality of life. Plus, for everything you avoid, there are hundreds of things to enjoy.

Guidelines for Eating

Every bit as important as what is eaten is how it is eaten. The manner in which we nourish ourselves can make a big difference in how we utilize the food we consume. There are a few guidelines which will make your dietary plan more healthful and enjoyable.

The most important principle of all is to eat in peace. To eat in a disrupted or agitated state is difficult on your body, regardless of the quality of the food you are eating. If you are unhappy or upset, wait until you are feeling better before eating. When you are in such a state, eating only puts a strain on the internal organs, which are already burdened by emotional stress.

Along the same lines is the idea that no matter what you eat, you should enjoy it. Maybe you will eat a pure, natural foods diet. On the other hand, maybe you will eat junk. But for your own inner well-being, enjoy yourself. Dont' lay guilt trips on yourself—it's fruitless. We're here to enjoy fulfillment and satisfaction, not to victimize ourselves with petty neurotic quirks, and this applies to eating as much as to anything else. The worst thing that you can do is tell yourself that you really shouldn't be eating something, and that by doing so you are going to get sick, or fat or whatever. If you choose to eat something in the first place, then don't complicate matters by telling yourself that you are committing a crime against your own health. The mind is so strong that such a way of thinking can easily become a self-fulfilling prophesy, and then what you eat really will make you sick. If you think you shouldn't eat something, then don't. Remember, you are in charge of yourself.

Chewing Food Thoroughly is a health practice that makes digestion a lot easier. The mouth is full of teeth which are designed to grind and tear foods. There are no teeth in the stomach, so all real breaking down of foods into small particles must be done in the mouth. Chew solid foods until they are liquefied. Not only does this make digestion much easier, but it also gives you an opportunity to more fully savor what you are eating. Chewing foods thoroughly brings out more of their flavor. Another thing that you will find is that if you chew thoroughly you will satisfy your hunger with less food. You will be less likely to overeat.

This brings us to the last guideline for eating, which is to avoid overeating. The body needs only a certain amount of food, and when you eat more than that, you strain the body rather than providing extra nourishment. Overeating is the main cause of obesity, which is a major health problem in the modern world. Though there is a lot of talk about "fat is beautiful" and "fat liberation," the truth is that being fat is a burden. Fat people live shorter lives and suffer from more chronic diseases than do those people of normal weight.

What is hardest on the body is going back and forth, losing and gaining weight over and over again. Studies now suggest that being either slightly overweight or slightly underweight is perfectly healthy. Bouncing up and down in weight puts stress on the system. People are likely to be healthiest by maintaining a steady weight through sensible eating habits and regular exercise. Systematic exercise promotes health and retards the aging process.

Also, your attitude toward food and life has a profound impact on your health. Food can be fun and a source of pleasure without being used as a security device or for emotional reassurance. If you eat sensibly, enjoy your food, and feel good about yourself in the process, you will remain healthy longer. The healthier you are, the more you can enjoy life and the opportunities that it offers.

The Yogatherapy Cleansing Program

The Yogatherapy Cleansing Program is a special program designed to cleanse the body of impurities which have built up over an extended period of time, and to rejuvenate the body by providing it with enzyme-rich foods which restore and build the vital life current within us. With this program, you can make significant positive gains in overall health and appearance. Digestion is enhanced, the skin begins to glow with the radiance of internal health, and energy increases. This program also enables you to benefit more fully from many of the Yogatherapy plans offered in the Yogatherapy Repertory.

The Yogatherapy Cleansing Program is a *40-day-raw-foods-plan* which utilizes fresh raw fruits, raw vegetables, fresh sprouted grains and seeds, and raw nuts only. All these foods are to be eaten in their whole, fresh and uncooked state, just as Nature grew them. I have seen hundreds of people on this raw foods diet, and the health benefits have been amazing. Often high blood pressure normalizes, arthritis clears up, allergies go away, energy increases, and there is greater mental alertness. You can remain on this diet for longer than 40 days if you wish, and many people do exactly that. However, if you live in a cold climate, it is best to limit the diet to 40 days, and then resume eating cooked grains and heavier foods for adequate body heat. Those who live in warm or tropical climates can follow the raw foods plan for years, if desired.

The Yogatherapy Cleansing Program includes a daily Yogatherapy exercise plan in addition to the diet. Each day the Yogatherapy routines for rejuvenation are done, along with *Soorya Namaskar* (Salute to the Sun). These allow the body to stretch, eliminate accumulated toxic waste products, and rejuvenate the glandular system. Through the Yogatherapy exercises and postures, circulation improves and overall stamina is increased. These along with the raw foods diet give the sparkling look and feel of health. When meditation is added to this regime, the combination is a superior formula for total well-being. Of course, just the diet alone will yield fine results, but the entire Yogatherapy Cleansing Program is a truly holistic approach.

The 40-day cleansing program begins with a 3-day-lemon-water-diet. For the first three days of the program, you consume only spring water with lemon in it. The ratio of water to lemon is about twelve ounces of water mixed with the juice of one fresh squeezed lemon. Bottled or presqueezed juices are not used. For these three days, no other food is consumed. At least eight glasses of lemon water should be drunk daily during this period, and you can drink more if you like. This has a strong cleansing effect. As lemon water passes through the alimentary tract, accumulated waste and mucus are drawn out of the body via the channels of elimination. The process is like an internal housecleaning, ridding the body of debris.

The upcoming section on fasting describes this process in more detail. It is important to note, though, that diabetics considering undertaking a fast should consult

104/Nutrition

a physician before doing so. Anyone with a serious health disorder would be well advised to do the same.

After the lemon water diet is done for a full three days, you move back to a solid food diet. This breaking of a fast is also described later in the section on fasting.

Cleansing Daily Schedule

A suggested plan to derive the maximum benefit from the 40-day-Yogatherapy-Cleansing-Program is as follows:

- Upon rising, brush your teeth, and then drink one large glass of lemon water. This is done every day, even after the 3-day-lemon-water-fast.
- Follow this with a hot shower, finished with a cold shower (see the section on hot and cold showers).
- Do your morning Yogatherapy exercise plan, consisting of the postures listed under Rejuvenation in the Yogatherapy Repertory.
- Relax for 5–10 minutes in Corpse Pose.
- Meditation 15–30 minutes (see Meditation).

Wait at least 15 minutes, and then eat breakfast, unless you are on the 3-day-lemon-water-fast. Breakfast will consist of fresh fruits, with fresh raw nuts and seeds if desired.

A typical breakfast might include a banana, an apple, and a handful of almonds or sunflower seeds, or a large, fresh fruit salad with nuts and berries.

Sometime between breakfast and lunch, be sure to drink one or two glasses of spring water. Lemon may be added if you like.

Lunch can be either a fruit meal or a vegetable meal. The vegetable lunch would be a salad made with fresh vegetables, sprouts of all kinds, lettuce, parsley, celery, spinach, tomatoes, and whatever you like. Avocados make a wonderful addition to salads, and sesame seeds or sunflower seeds can be added for protein. The ideal salad dressing is made with equal parts of virgin olive oil and fresh lemon juice, to which some ground cayenne, kelp powder, and ground herbs can be added for additional flavor.

Again, between lunch and dinner drink one or two glasses of spring water or lemon water.

Supper is another vegetable salad. You will learn to be creative with salads as you go, adding shredded radish, chopped raw beets, sliced zucchini, avocados, nuts and seeds, as you concoct a variety of different raw vegetable repasts. You can also grind nuts and seeds in a blender with the olive oil and lemon juice dressing, making a creamier, nutty salad dressing.

In the evening, at least three or more hours after eating, again do Salute to the Sun and the Rejuvenation Series from Chapter II, if you can make the time. Follow this with a meditation. This will top off your day with energy, peace, and a sense of inner balance. Sleep will be deeper and more satisfying, and you will feel fresher in the morning, when you start the day again.

You may have to modify this suggested schedule to suit your own needs and activities. If you usually eat only twice a day, then omit one of the meals. Or perhaps you would like to substitute fresh juices for a solid meal. In any case, try to avoid snacking, as the cleansing program is designed to give your body a break, and snacking will work against that goal.

To enable you to be more imaginative in preparing enjoyable raw foods meal while on the Yogatherapy cleansing diet, the following books will be helpful for recipes.

Love Your Body, by Viktoras Kulvinskas
Cookin' with Mother Nature, by Dick Gregory
Light Eating for Survival, by Marcia Acciardo

Please be advised that the authors of the above books believe that the raw foods diet is the only healthful diet. As a result, the books contain extreme dietary philosophies which are quite biased. But if you overlook those shortcomings, the recipes can be of great value.

You can expect several things from the Yogatherapy Cleansing Program. For the first three days you will probably be hungry, especially if you are not used to fasting. Once you are on solid foods, the daily plan will likely be very different than what you are used to following. Most people lose some weight, and for everyone the diet takes getting adjusted. But after a few days, you should be well into the swing of things. Please do yourself a favor though—don't loiter around the kitchen, and try not to become totally preoccupied with food. Just eat when you need to, and then carry on with the rest of your daily schedule. By following the exercise plan every day you will become stronger, more flexible, and more energetic. You will find it easier to relax, and your sleep will be more satisfying as well.

During the cleansing program, the liver and the intestines will start to detoxify, and old waste matter will be expelled from the body. As this process begins, you may temporarily feel weak. Then again, you may not. Sometimes weakness is caused by extra circulation of toxic wastes in the body as they start to be eliminated. This fatigue is temporary, though, and can be lessened by maintaining a high water intake. Some people also experience a temporary outbreak of pimples during cleansing. This also is a result of detoxification, and while it is annoying, it will go away. Many people feel great from the very first day of the cleansing program, without fatigue or signs of detoxification. But you should be aware of these possible discomforts, so that you understand what is going on with your body.

After the 40-day-Yogatherapy-Cleansing-Program, you may want to reintroduce a broader range of foods to your diet. To explore the most healthful and tasteful variety of foods, the following cookbooks will be valuable.

Natural Foods Cookbook, by Mary Estella
Ten Talents, by Frank and Rosalie Hurd
Recipes for a Small Planet, by Ellen Buchman Ewald

The Book of Whole Meals, by Annemarie Colbin
Laurel's Kitchen, by Robertson, Laurel
Tassajara Cooking, by Edward Espe Brown
The Deaf Smith Country Cookbook, by Ford, Hillyard, and Koock

Because diet is a factor essential to good health, it is worth while to learn about food and nutrition, and how what you eat affects the way that you think and feel. The Yogatherapy diet and the Yogatherapy cleansing program will enable you to get more out of life, by providing your body with wholesome, vital nutrition. In combination with the Yogatherapy exercises and postures, your dietary plan will work for your extended health and vitality. The Yoga techniques are so powerful that as you embark upon your Yogatherapy program, a revolution will begin to occur in your body/mind.

Super Foods

While there are thousands of wholesome, nutritious foods in the world, there are some that are so rich in nutrients that they are known as super foods. The following is a list of some superfoods, virtually all of which are commonly available. Added to your diet, these superfoods can significantly enhance your nutritional status.

Alfalfa: One of the heartiest of all plants, alfalfa sinks its roots dozens of feet into the ground, drawing up precious minerals and trace elements into the leaves of this nutrient-rich crop. Alfalfa is high in minerals and trace elements, high in carotenes (natural pro-vitamin A), rich in chlorophyll, a good source of vitamin K, and high in fiber. Alfalfa also contains stigmasterol, known as the "anti-stiffness factor," which is of value in the treatment of arthritis. Alfalfa is available in tablet form, which is a convenient way to eat this nutritious crop.

Almonds: Often referred to as the "King of Nuts," almonds are high in riboflavin, protein, vitamin E and calcium. Almonds have been used for centuries by the Hindus, Arabs and Chinese as an aid to sexual potency. The *Ayurveda*, India's classical Hindu health text, states that almonds are good for the brain, and that their oil replenishes spinal fluid.

Apples: This common fruit is excellent for digestion, and is of value for people with sensitive stomachs. Apples are useful in cases of dysentery and diarrhea. They are high in potassium, sulfur, and silicon. Apple pectin rids the body of toxic wastes, and reduces blood cholesterol.

Avocados: The name of this rich fruit comes from the Aztec word for testicle, due to its appearance as it hangs from the tree. High in protein, vitamin A, potassium, and essential fatty acids, this highly concentrated food is used as a meat substitute. It is eaten mainly in salads, where it is chopped plain or served mashed as guacamole. There are hundreds of varieties of avocados, the richest of which is the Haas variety grown in California.

Bananas: High in potassium, magnesium, and phosphorous, bananas are also rich in natural sugars. They are ideal high energy foods, and the *Ayurveda* considers bananas to be rejuvenators and aphrodisiac. Due to their high sugar content, they should be avoided by people with blood sugar disorders or obesity. Otherwise, bananas are good food, and are easy to digest, provided that the peels are spotted, to indicate full ripeness.

Bee Pollen: Gathered by bees from the mature stamens of flower blossoms, bee pollen is a complete protein, and contains vitamins A, the B-complex, C, D, E, and K. It is rich in minerals and is naturally antibiotic. Pollen is widely used by athletes to increase endurance and stamina. It is of value in the treatment of anemia, constipation, flatulence, and general weakness. Although pollen comes in many forms, the best is fresh-refrigerated, if you can get it.

Beets: A valuable source of potassium, chlorine, and silicon, beets are a powerful energy food. They are excellent for digestion, and are useful in combatting weakness, fatigue, and constipation. Beets are valuable for cleansing the liver. Raw beets are very powerful, and should be eaten sparingly, as they can stimulate very rapid intestinal activity.

Bran: Wheat bran, oat bran, and rice bran are all high in B-vitamins, but are best known as high fiber foods. All three add to intestinal bulk, thereby enhancing elimination. Wheat bran is the most vigorous of the three for speeding up intestinal motility. Many people find that they prefer to use oat bran or rice bran instead. A generous intake of bran, along with a good natural diet, is an effective preventive measure against gallstones, hemorrhoids, constipation, diverticulitis, and many other metabolic disorders.

Brown Rice: While rice is a staple grain in most Asian and Oriental countries, usually the rice eaten is white rice, of which the bran and germ layers have been stripped away. The process of making white rice robs most of the nutrients from the grain. Brown rice, on the other hand, is a superbly concentrated food, the nutrients of which remain intact. The cult philosophy of Macrobiotics considers brown rice to be not only the ultimate food, but the key to saving the world as well. While this is excessive, it is true that brown rice fortifies the body, strengthens the digestive organs, and is an excellent food for slow, steady energy production. Combined with beans, brown rice forms a complete protein. Brown rice will store for generations, and people have recovered from a variety of health disorders by including regular portions of brown rice in their diets.

Buttermilk: This is one of the easiest to digest of all milk products. Buttermilk is useful for those suffering from weight loss and weakness, it enhances digestion, and is strengthening. The juice of ginger root can be added to buttermilk for those who suffer from very poor digestion and weakness.

Chilis: These are hot peppers, all of which are members of the capsicum family. Chilis are very high in natural vitamin A, and are best known for their hot taste. There are many varieties of chilis, whose temperatures range from mildly warm to blazing hot. Chilis stimulate digestion, appetite, and bowel activity. They help to rid the body of accumulated mucous and internal debris, and thus are effective as cleansers. Chilis can be used fresh, or dried and powdered. If you are not used to eating chilis, start out slowly. They can burn twice, going into your body, and coming out. Chilis are valuable for people with sinus congestion, poor circulation, constipation, and headaches.

Cod Liver Oil: In spite of its disagreeable taste, cod liver oil is an excellent all-natural source of vitamins A and D. Vitamin A builds resistance to infection, promotes growth and vitality, is necessary for pregnancy and lactation, for good vision and night sight, and helps the growth, maintenance, and repair of healthy skin and lining tissues, hair, teeth, bones, and glands. Vitamin D is involved in the utilization of calcium and phosphorous, proper formation of bones and teeth, and for healthy skin. Cod liver oil is not only excellent for humans, but is valuable for cats and dogs, helping to prevent dry, scaling skin, and producing a glowing coat of fur.

Garlic: Widely used in Oriental and Indian medicines, garlic is a treasured healing agent. Though best known for its powerful aroma and flavor in the preparation of foods, garlic is also a powerful antibiotic, and is often referred to as "Russian Penicillin," as it has been widely used in Russian clinics. Garlic is antibacterial, is a blood purifier, and is aphrodisiac. It is used to treat all respiratory problems, blood-pressure disorders, poor digestion, intestinal gas, skin diseases, tumors, kidney trouble, liver disorders, bladder infections, colds, and flu.

Ginger Root: Another spice used widely in Asia, the Orient, and tropical islands, ginger root stimulates appetite and promotes perspiration. It is used for colds, flu, and digestive disorders, and is usually boiled in water and drunk as a tea. Ginger root, in tea or capsule form, is also very effective for motion sickness, and is more valuable than most nonprescription remedies for the same thing.

Honey: Sometimes referred to as the "Nectar of the Gods," honey is a sweet elixir made by bees from the nectar of flowers. There are hundreds of flavors of honeys, made from various blossoms. The only honey worth eating is raw, unfiltered honey. Such honey is rich in enzymes and minerals, B-vitamins, and some vitamin C. Honey is a first-class restorative, and is mixed with heated milk and the juice of ginger root in the treatment of poor digestion, weakness, and debility.

Kelp: This is a seaweed which grows in huge beds, like underwater forests. Kelp beds are found off the coasts of California, Norway, Japan, and other parts of the world. Because kelp is a sea vegetable which grows in seawater, it is rich in minerals and trace elements. At least 72 of these are found in kelp, though kelp is best known for its iodine value. Kelp is of value to digestion, healthy hair, skin, nails, bones and teeth. It is useful for overall health and vitality. Due to its iodine content, kelp is valuable to the thyroid gland, which regulates metabolism. In quantity, kelp tablets help sluggish bowels to function properly.

Lecithin: This natural substance is found in virtually every one of the body's 60 trillion cells. Lecithin is found in almost every food known, but is concentrated in soybeans, eggs, and liver. Soybeans are the common commercial source of lecithin, which is necessary for maintaining health, for the metabolism of fats, and for maximizing the effectiveness of vitamins A, D, and E. Lecithin has been shown to reduce serum cholesterol, dissolve arterial plaque, and lower blood pressure. Phosphatidyl choline, a substance found in quantity in lecithin, produces acetylcholine, a brain chemical which functions in memory and mental clarity. Lecithin granules or high phosphatidyl choline capsules are the best ways to take this superfood.

Nutritional Yeast: Commonly known as brewer's yeast, nutritional yeast is a particular strain of yeast (*saccharomyces cerevisiae*) which is grown for nutritional purposes. Nutritional yeast has three outstanding virtues. The first is that it is a good source of natural B-vitamins. Thus yeast is a good food for enhancing digestive and nerve function, growth and vitality. Secondly, yeast is a good source of protein. At about 54% protein, yeast makes an excellent protein supplement. Thirdly, nutritional yeast is easy to digest. Thus the carbohydrate, protein, and B-vitamin value is available to the body readily, without much effort on the part of the digestive system.

Olive Oil: Olive oil is the most nutritious and most easily digested vegetable oil. Unheated, it will store for long periods without turning rancid. Rich in essential fatty acids, olive oil provides important nutrients for healthy skin, hair, sex organs, hormone production, nerves, and circulation. Virgin olive oil, the very first oil to drip from olives at the commencement of pressing, is preferred over all other varieties. Greeks drink a mouthful of olive oil followed by a spoonful of raw honey first thing in the morning to flush out the bile ducts and feed the sex organs. Virgin olive oil can be used liberally, as it is one of the most health-bestowing foods known.

Papaya: This tropical fruit is sweet, nutritious, and very easy to digest. Papayas contain papain, a powerful protein-digesting enzyme. Thus papaya is valuable for digesting protein foods. It is also useful for helping to eat up mucus in the digestive tract, as mucus is a protein substance. Papaya is one of the only two sweet fruits that can be eaten with heavy protein foods. Papain is used commercially as the principle agent in commercial meat tenderizers.

110/NUTRITION

Pineapple: This tropical fruit is the other sweet fruit that can be eaten with heavy protein foods. Pineapple also contains a protein-digesting enzyme, bromelain, which aids in the digestion of proteins, and also helps to clean debris from the digestive tract. Bromelain is also an anti-inflammatory substance, and is used pharmaceutically in the treatment of inflammation of many kinds, including arthritis.

Sesame: Sesame has been so highly regarded that in some cultures it has been credited with mystical powers. Thus the term "open sesame." This seed contains ample quantities of calcium and vitamin E, and is recommended in the *Ayurveda* as a restorative and sexual food. The oil of sesame is reputed to be good for the brain, and this remarkable seed is a staple food in many middle-Eastern nations, due to its high protein value.

Sushi/Sashimi: *Sushi* is a Japanese specialty food, consisting of a strip of raw fish laid on top of a small log of rice. *Sashimi* is the raw fish without the rice. Though many Westerners initially recoil at the idea of eating raw fish, *sushi* and *sashimi* have become very popular foods recently, due to their exceptional taste and their high nutrient value. Fresh, raw fish is high in protein, vitamins, and minerals, is generally low in fat, and is easy to digest. It is strengthening, and valuable for people who suffer from weakness, fatigue, or poor digestion. *Sushi* and *sashimi* are considered by some people to be aphrodisiac, as they can enhance sexual function. Raw fish is not only a wonderful taste treat, but is excellent nutrition as well.

Sprout Chart

Fresh sprouts are excellent foods, high in vitamins and live enzymes. While sprouts can be purchased, they can also be grown at home. The following chart is for growing sprouts by the jar method. Using either a quart or gallon size jar, soak your sprout seeds for 6 hours, as indicated. Then drain the water. Cover the top of your jar with gauze, secured with an elastic band, and keep the jar at a slant, to allow for continuous drainage and circulation of air. Rinse your sprouts with fresh water at least two times daily. For the last day of growth, expose your sprouts to plenty of light, so that they will become green with natural chlorophyll. Drain your sprouts completely before harvesting them, and keep them refrigerated in an airtight container.

Seed	Amount	Soaking Time	Harvest Time
Alfalfa	1 tbsp./Qt.–3 tbsp./Gal.	6 hours	5–7 days
Fenugreek	2 tbsp./Qt.–4 tbsp./Gal.	6 hours	5–7 days
Radish	1 tbsp./Qt.–3 tbsp./Gal.	6 hours	3–4 days
Red Clover	1 tbsp./Qt.–3 tbsp./Gal.	6 hours	5–7 days
Lentil	1/4th jar of seed	6 hours	5–7 days
Sunflower	1/4th jar of seed	6 hours	1 1/2–2 days
Mung Bean	1/4th jar of seed	6 hours	3–4 days
Whole Wheat	2 tbsp./Qt.–4 tbsp./Gal.	6 hours	3–4 days

For further sprouting information, see *The Sprout Book*, by Viktoras Kulvinskas.

Wheat Germ and Wheat Germ Oil: The germ layer of the whole wheat kernel is a concentrated source of B-vitamins, minerals, and vitamin E. Per gram weight, wheat germ is one of the most nutritious cereal foods known. It is an excellent energy food. The oil pressed from wheat germ contains a substance known as *octacosanol*, which has been proven to increase muscular strength, and enhance stamina and endurance. Octacosanol has also demonstrated therapeutic value in the treatment of some neuromuscular disorders. Both wheat germ and wheat germ oil are concentrated foods that can be eaten by anyone wanting more nutrition, energy, power, and stamina.

Yogurt: A cultured milk product, yogurt is made with friendly bacteria which are beneficial to the intestines. These bacteria enhance intestinal activity, and also stimulate the internal production of B-vitamins. The bacteria consume unfriendly microbes, and help to prevent over acidity in the bowels. Yogurt is high in protein, is easy to digest, enhances bowel regularity, and provides calcium.

Fasting

Of all of Nature's ways to heal the body, one of the most effective is fasting. When the body is not fed solid foods, all the energy which normally goes to digestion is instead used for self regeneration. Over the course of a fast there is great cleansing taking place. Toxic waste, mucus, and accumulated debris such as dead cells are eliminated from the body. As this happens, there is less stress on the body, and the process of regeneration can begin. Internal organs regain their proper integrity, shape, and function, and their tissue becomes strong and healthy. The complexion clears, excess weight is lost, energy increases, and there is internal and external cleanliness. Fasting is natural. When animals are sick, they fast instinctively.

There are many different ways to fast. The most common fast is a water fast, during which one drinks water only. No solid or liquid foods are taken during this time. A plain water fast can last from one day to even a couple of weeks. A water fast is certainly the simplest, and certainly the most austere of all fasts.

During a water fast it is essential to make sure that you drink copious amounts of water. You should manage to drink at least ten or more glasses a day. This is necessary in order to eliminate waste materials. Without ample fluid in the system the body will start to circulate toxic waste right into the bloodstream. This can lead to autointoxication, or self poisoning. Many people who have died from "hunger" have actually succumbed to an excess of toxins in the bloodstream while fasting involuntarily due to some extreme condition such as a natural disaster. It takes a long time for the average healthy person to die of hunger, but one can die of self poisoning rather quickly. It is imperative, then, to consume large amounts of water while on a water fast.

However, a plain water fast is not necessarily the best or most effective fast. I personally believe that a lemon water fast, as described in the Yogatherapy Cleansing Program, is superior. Lemon provides essential vitamins and minerals, and is a powerful detoxifying agent. The same rules which apply to a water fast apply to a lemon water fast. You should drink a lot every day that you fast, in order to enable your body to effectively eliminate waste matter.

While fasting it is important to bathe regularly, both to stimulate circulation and to keep the body clean. When you fast, a lot of elimination takes place through the pores of the skin. Thus bathing is necessary to assist in total cleansing. It is beneficial to use a loofa sponge on the whole body, scrubbing the skin until it glows. This will greatly improve surface circulation, and will massage natural oils back into the skin.

There are a couple of points worth making here. One is that if you are going to undertake a fast for longer than ten days, you would be well advised to seek expert supervision. Get in touch with a naturopathic doctor or someone who is experienced in supervising a fast. I would advise this for anyone who has no fasting experience, because fasting is a science in itself, and a knowledgeable person can be of great value to you.

Breaking a fast is very, very important. This cannot be emphasized strongly enough. You must always break a fast on light foods, in small quantities. For every three days that you have fasted on liquids, you should eat only fresh, easy to digest raw fruits for one day. So a six day lemon water fast would be followed by two days of eating fruit. If a fast is broken improperly, all hell can break loose. One woman I know broke a 27-day-fast on pizza and corn bread, and was seriously sick for four months as a result. If you choose to fast, break the fast properly.

Enemas are often taken during a fast. There is some controversy as to whether or not enemas should be used to assist cleansing. About this I can only say that from what I have seen, enemas are definitely helpful during a fast. They assist and speed up internal cleansing. They are safe and effective, and are therefore advisable. On a fast, you will get better results if an enema or colonic irrigation is taken at least once a day. A fast will be of value with or without the internal bathing provided by enemas, but enemas do rid the bowels of accumulated waste quickly. However, enemas are not to be used regularly when one is on a solid food diet. This tends to make one dependant upon them for normal bowel activity.

Another type of fast which is popular and highly effective is the juice fast. Basically a juice fast utilizes the cleansing and rebuilding properties of various fresh vegetable and fruit juices. Many health experts feel that juice fasting is the best, most effective type of fast. Juices are more satisfying than water or lemon water, and they do provide a lot of concentrated nourishment.

For serious, degenerative conditions the most comprehensive juice program is the one developed by Dr. Max Gerson. Known simply as the Gerson Therapy, it has been highly successful in the treatment and cure of several types of cancer. The book *A Cancer Therapy, Results of Fifty Cases*, carefully describes the Gerson Therapy. The program has proven beneficial to individuals with other very serious health disorders besides cancer.

A good book on juice fasting is Dr. Paavo Airola's book *How to Keep Slim, Healthy and Young with Juice Fasting*. For a more detailed account of the lemon water diet, see Stanley Burrough's book *Healing for the Age of Enlightenment*. And for some excellent insights into fasting in general, see Prof. Arnold Ehret's book *Rational Fasting*.

Juices, How to Prepare Them

Juices are most healthful when drunk fresh, immediately after juicing. If juices sit, even for half an hour, they rapidly lose nutrients, due to exposure to oxygen. Thus you are advised to drink your juices fresh, just as soon as you extract them. For this you will need to purchase a juice extractor. Juicers are worthwhile investments, and will provide you with the means to make your own fresh juices daily.

If you need to take juice to work, or will be in a situation in which you cannot make your juice and drink it immediately, then carry your juices in a clean, airtight container, and do not overexpose them to either heat or light. Refrigeration will keep juices fresh longer.

Juices are highly concentrated foods. Do not gulp them down. Drink juices slowly, and swish them around in your mouth. Juices must be thoroughly insalivated to digest thoroughly and quickly. They should mix with your saliva, just as though they were solid foods.

Juice/Ailment Chart

For every health disorder, there are corresponding nutritional factors. There are many ways to work with these factors, one of which is to utilize the concentrated nutritional value of fresh juices. The following chart is a list of ailments and juice formulas recommended for each one. While it is not legal to claim any direct therapeutic benefits from juices or juice formulas, it is worthy of note that fresh juices can enhance a person's nutritional status, which in turn supports the body's own innate capacity for self-healing. Most formulas listed make a twelve ounce drink, which can be taken one or more times daily. You will need to experiment to determine what total amount of daily juice intake is appropriate for you.

Acidosis: carrot 8 oz., spinach 4 oz.
Acne: carrot 6 oz., spinach 4 oz., parsley 2 oz.
Adenoids: carrot 10 oz., parsley 2 oz., 2 cloves garlic (leave out garlic if formula is given to children)
Allergies: carrot 8 oz., cucumber 2 oz., beet 2 oz.
Anemia: carrot 6 oz., beet 3 oz., spinach 3 oz.

Arterial Disease: celery 4 oz., spinach 4 oz., lettuce 2 oz., parsley 2 oz.
Arthritis: carrot 8 oz., spinach 4 oz., or, grapefruit 6 oz., celery 6 oz.
Asthma: carrot 8 oz., radish 2 oz., lemon 2 oz.
Bladder Disorders: carrot 4 oz., celery 4 oz., spinach 4 oz.
Blood Pressure, High: carrot 6 oz., spinach 4 oz., parsley 2 oz., garlic, 2 cloves.
Blood Pressure, Low: carrot 8 oz., cucumber 2 oz., beet 2 oz.
Bronchitis: carrot 8 oz., radish 2 oz., lemon 2 oz.
Bursitis: carrot 8 oz., spinach 4 oz., or, pineapple 6 oz., celery 6 oz.
Catarrh: celery 6 oz., spinach 4 oz., radish 2 oz., with optional garlic, 2 cloves.
Colds: 1 fresh lemon in hot water, with garlic, 2 cloves, or, celery 6 oz., radish 4 oz., lemon 2 oz.
Colitis: carrot 8 oz., cucumber 2 oz., beet 2 oz.
Constipation: apple 8 oz., spinach 4 oz., or, carrot 6 oz., beet 3 oz., spinach 3 oz.
Cystitis: carrot 4 oz., celery 4 oz., spinach 4 oz.
Diarrhea: celery 6 oz., spinach 2 oz., lettuce 2 oz., parsley 2 oz.
Dysentery: carrot 6 oz., celery 6 oz., garlic, 2 cloves.
Eczema: celery 4 oz., spinach 4 oz., lettuce 2 oz., parsley 2 oz.
Fatigue: carrot 6 oz., beet 4 oz., parsley 2 oz.
Gallbladder, Gallstones: carrot 6 oz., cucumber 2 oz., beet 2 oz., parsley 2 oz.
Gout: celery 4 oz., spinach 4 oz., lettuce 2 oz., parsley 2 oz.
Halitosis: carrot 6 oz., spinach 4 oz., parsley 2 oz.
Hay Fever: celery 4 oz., spinach 4 oz., parsley 2 oz., radish 2 oz.
Headaches: carrot 6 oz., spinach 4 oz., parsley 2 oz.
Heart Disease: carrot 6 oz., beet 2 oz., celery 4 oz.
Hemorrhoids: carrot 6 oz., spinach 4 oz., parsley 2 oz.
Indigestion: pineapple or, pineapple 8 oz., ginger 1 oz., or, celery 6 oz., spinach 4 oz., parsley 2 oz.
Influenza: celery 6 oz., radish 4 oz., lemon 2 oz.
Insomnia: celery 4 oz., spinach 4 oz., lettuce 2 oz., parsley 2 oz.
Kidney Disorders: carrot 4 oz., celery 4 oz., spinach 4 oz.
Liver Disorders: carrot 8 oz., beet 4 oz.
Menopause: celery 4 oz., spinach 4 oz., lettuce 2 oz., parsley 2 oz.
Nervous Disorders: celery 6 oz., beet 3 oz., parsley 2 oz., ginger 1 oz.
Obesity: grapefruit or, celery 8 oz., parsley 2 oz., lemon 2 oz.
Pneumonia: celery 6 oz., radish 2 oz., parsley 2 oz., lemon 2 oz.
Prostate Disorders: carrot 4 oz., celery 4 oz., spinach 4 oz.
Pyorrhea: carrot 4 oz., celery 4 oz., parsley 2 oz., spinach 2 oz.
Rheumatism: carrot 8 oz., spinach 4 oz., or, pineapple 6 oz., celery 6 oz.
Sinus Disorders: celery 6 oz., spinach 3 oz., radish 3 oz.
Tonsillitis: carrot 10 oz., parsley 2 oz., garlic, 2 cloves (leave out garlic if formula is given to children)
Toxemia: carrot 4 oz., celery 4 oz., parsley 2 oz., spinach 2 oz.
Ulcers: carrot 6 oz., cucumber 4 oz., spinach 2 oz.
Varicose Veins: carrot 6 oz., green pepper 4 oz., parsley 2 oz.

VITAMINS, MINERALS, and FOOD SUPPLEMENTS

Vitamins, Minerals, and Food Supplements

One very significant component of the Yogatherapy approach to health is the judicious use of vitamins, minerals, and assorted food supplements. These are recommended to enhance nutritional status, and to provide essential materials for a variety of physiological functions.

One current point of view is that we should be able to obtain all the nutrients we need from the foods we eat, and that therefore all food supplements are unnecessary. It would be wonderful if we could in fact obtain all the nutrients we need from the foods we eat. However, there are several reasons why this is not feasible:

Depleted Soil: The soil in major agricultural areas in the United States and other developed nations has quickly become deficient in the nutrients essential to the growth of nutritious foods. Because the soil in most agricultural areas is nutrient poor, the foods grown in that soil are nutrient poor as well.

Transit Time and Storage: Most people purchase their foods from grocery stores, rather than simply stepping out into the back yard and picking, or slaughtering, whatever they need. When food is sold in stores, it has been picked, packed, cooled, stored, shipped, distributed, stored, displayed, and then sold. During the time between picking (or slaughtering) and actual consumption of food, many nutrients are lost. Time, heat, light, and moisture are all destroyers of vitamins.

Processing: With the exception of some vegetables, fruits, grains, beans, and nuts, most foods go through some sort of processing, by which they are altered for purposes of flavor, appearance, and shelf life. During processing, many nutrients are lost. Even when foods are refortified, their original nutritional value is not duplicated.

Cooking: Most people cook their food. While this is perfectly desirable, it is also true that some nutrients are lost during cooking.

The above factors have to do with why foods do not actually contain what they are supposed to. However, there are still other reasons to consume vitamins and food supplements:

Poor Dietary Intake: Most people do not eat a diet consisting only of nutritious, high quality foods. Thus the nutrient value of the average person's total dietary intake could be much higher. It is estimated that 95% of the American public is marginally deficient in at least one of six major nutrients, directly due to dietary intake.

Chemicals in Foods (Agricultural): Toxic chemicals are commonly used in agriculture and livestock production. Fertilizers, pesticides, fungicides, dusts, sprays, waxes, hormones, and antibiotics occur in foods, due to their commercial use in food production. These chemicals diminish nutrient levels in the body.

Chemical Additives (Food Processing): Other toxic chemicals are frequently employed in the processing of foods. Over 400 commonly used chemicals are currently under investigation as possible cancer causing agents. These food processing chemicals include preservatives, artificial flavoring, and artificial coloring. These also diminish nutrient levels in the body.

Stresses: To a great extent, we are unnatural people living in an unnatural world. There are innumerable stresses, from commuting, to noise pollution, to air pollution, to schedule pressures, which all diminish the body's stores of nutrients.

In addition to all of the above factors, each person is biochemically unique. Thus some people need as much as several hundred times the intake of certain nutrients as other people do. Often, such amounts of nutrients are not readily obtainable in reasonable quantities of foods. For all of the above reasons, nutritional supplementation is acceptable, desirable, and necessary.

All Supplements Are Not Alike: The quality of vitamins and food supplements varies greatly from brand to brand. Typically, drug store and mail order brands tend to be of poor quality, and unreliable potency. Overall, the brands available at natural food stores are higher quality, and use better materials. However, don't be fooled by brands which claim to be "all natural," or "organic." Vitamins are manufactured from highly refined pharmaceutical raw materials. They are not squeezed from fruits and vegetables, as some companies suggest. Nonetheless, vitamins are biologically active, and they do enhance the millions of various bodily functions which are dependant upon nutrients. My recommendation is to purchase only those brands which offer freshness dating on the label, which guarantee potency, which have good reputations, and which will supply you with technical information if you need it.

How and When to Take Supplements: Supplements are exactly what the name implies—they are supplementary to a good diet. For best assimilation and utilization, they should be taken with meals. With the exception of vitamin C, vitamins shouldn't be taken on an empty stomach, and should not be taken while fasting.

The RDA = Recommended Dietary Allowances

The RDA—What Are They?

"The RDA are recommendations for the average daily amounts of nutrients that population groups should consume over a period of time." This statement, made in the Ninth Edition of the Recommended Dietary Allowances, expresses the intent of the Food and Nutrition Board of the National Academy of Sciences. This board establishes the RDA for Energy, Carbohydrates, Fiber, Fat, Protein, Vitamins, Minerals, Trace Elements, Water and Electrolytes. These recommendations are the accepted national standard in the United States for nutrient intake. For this reason, they are of concern to anyone truly interested in nutrition.

How Are the RDA Determined?

According to the Food and Nutrition Board of the National Academy of Science, a number of techniques are employed to arrive at the RDA. These techniques include the following:

1. Collection of data on nutrient intake from the food supply of apparently normal, healthy people.
2. Review of epidemiological observations when clinical consequences of nutrient deficiencies are found to be correctable by dietary improvement.
3. Biochemical measurements that assess degree of tissue saturation or adequacy of molecular function in relation to nutrient intake.
4. Nutrient balance studies that measure nutritional status in relation to intake.
5. Studies of subjects maintained on diets containing marginally low or deficient levels of a nutrient, followed by correction of the deficit with measured amounts of that nutrient.
6. Extrapolation from animal experiments in which deficiencies have been produced by the exclusion of a single nutrient from the diet.

While these methods are well intended, there is a basic error underlying the entire approach. This error is found in the first method used to determine the RDA: "collection of data on nutrient intake from the food supply of apparently normal, healthy people."

The term "apparently normal, healthy people" is vague and ambiguous at best, and is open to the widest possible interpretation. Health means different things to different people. To many, the absence of serious disease is health. To others, health is a vital, dynamic condition. To the Food and Nutrition Board, health, as it pertains to the evaluation of nutrient status, is a condition in which there are no detectable signs of clinical deficiencies, and no serious pathologies such as cancer, emphysema, or heart disease. In other words, health in this instance is the absence of clinical conditions.

The deficiency condition associated with inadequate dietary vitamin C intake is scurvy. The symptoms of scurvy include lassitude, weakness, irritability, weight loss, swollen gums which become split and spongy, loosening of teeth, spontaneous hemorrhages, and other phenomena. The end result of scurvy is death. Any of the above signs would be looked for in the evaluation process of the RDA, and would suffice to exclude a person from the study.

But the above signs are not the *only* symptoms of vitamin C deficiency. They are the *clinical* signs. A number of distinguished nutritional scientists (including Dr. Roger Williams, Dr. Linus Pauling, and Dr. Jeffrey Bland) insist that there are also many *subclinical* deficiency symptoms as well. Susceptibility to the common cold may be a sign of inadequate dietary vitamin C intake. The Food and Nutrition Board does not exclude from its surveys individuals who suffer from colds.

Nor are borderline hypoglycemics, allergy sufferers, individuals with occasional fatigue, gas, insomnia, menstrual cramps, or acne excluded from the studies. Yet all of these problems may be nutritionally related, though they are not considered in the estimation of the RDA. Essentially, then, a great deal of data used to determine the RDA is obtained from the study of individuals who may have any of hundreds of subclinical nutrient deficiencies.

In light of this unfortunate fact, one can only conclude that the RDA are insufficient standards for dietary intake. However, there is more to the story.

Biochemical Individuality

Biochemical individuality is the biological and chemical uniqueness of each person. Though a healthy person will have two eyes, a nose, a mouth, and four limbs, there are variations in height, weight, skeletal structure, hair and skin color, and hundreds of other known factors. Just as with fingerprints, no two people are truly alike. Truly, similarities do exist—but everyone is in fact different.

The RDA, however, give extremely little allowance for such differences between people, and assign identical nutrient requirements to highly differentiated groups. For example, according to the RDA, pregnant women, elementary school children, and 20 years old athletes all have the same vitamin C requirements. Supposedly they all need 60 milligrams of vitamin C daily. Does this make any sense to you?

According to the RDA, 12 years old girls, 45 years old executive males, and 85 years old grandmothers all require 1.5 milligrams of thiamine daily.

If adequate nutritional status is a goal in the establishment of the RDA, then these standards must reflect a profound understanding of biochemical variances in the human species. However, no such understanding is either stated or implied. As a result, the RDA are a poor, inadequate group of standards geared toward nutritional mediocrity. This is certainly not intentional—but it is certainly the case.

What Does This Mean?

Some individuals may require gram quantities of vitamin C daily, while others may function well on a fraction of that amount. Equally large variations exist for pantothenic acid, other B-vitamins, iron, and other nutrients. Because there are such variations in human nutritional needs, there must be a wide range of supplement products to choose from. For this reason, vitamin and mineral products are available in many potencies, from conservative amounts to mega-doses. A product with several thousand percent of the RDA may be unnecessary for some people, but exactly appropriate for others.

In this book some guidelines are given for suggested dosage amounts of nutrients. However, each individual is different. You will need to experiment with yourself to determine what is optimal for you.

United States Recommended Dietary Allowances for the 12 Essential Vitamins and the 7 Essential Minerals

	Children 12 months to four years old	Adults and Children four years or older	Pregnant or Lactating Women
Vitamin A	2,500 I.U.	5,000 I.U.	8,000 I.U.
Vitamin D	400 I.U.	400 I.U.	400 I.U.
Vitamin E	10 I.U.	30 I.U.	30 I.U.
Vitamin C	40 mg.	60 mg.	60 mg.
Folic Acid	0.2 mg.	0.4 mg.	0.8 mg.
Thiamine (B_1)	0.7 mg.	1.5 mg.	1.7 mg.
Riboflavin (B_2)	0.8 mg.	1.7 mg.	2.0 mg.
Niacin	9 mg.	20 mg.	20 mg.
Vitamin B_6	0.7 mg.	2.0 mg.	2.5 mg.
Vitamin B_{12}	3 mcg.	6 mcg.	8 mcg.
Biotin	0.15 mg.	0.3 mg.	0.3 mg.
Pantothenic Acid	5 mg.	10 mg.	10 mg.
Calcium	0.8 gm.	1 gm.	1.3 gm.
Phosphorous	0.8 gm.	1 gm.	1.3 gm.
Iodine	70 mcg.	150 mcg.	150 mcg.
Iron	10 mg.	18 mg.	18 mg.
Magnesium	200 mg.	400 mg.	450 mg.
Copper	1 mg.	2 mg.	2 mg.
Zinc	8 mg.	15 mg.	15 mg.

The Nutrient Section

The format of this Nutrient Section is designed for quick, easy access to basic information pertaining to a total of thirty vitamins and minerals. For each nutrient, six categories of information are provided. The following explanations of these categories will enable you to best understand the material given in this section.

Sources: For each nutrient, the best food sources are given. A broad range of choices is listed whenever possible. However, fortified foods such as enriched cereals, breads, and other packaged of processed items, are not listed. The given sources selection is based on the vitamin and mineral values of whole foods, or their non-fortified products, such as dairy items and vegetable oils. In most cases, there are other sources for the nutrients than the ones listed. These, however, usually contain insignificant quantities of a particular nutrient, and are therefore not worthy of mention.

Known Functions: Inasmuch as nutrition is a variable and non-exact science at this point in time, you must understand that there are ten times as many unknowns as there are knowns with regard to vitamins and minerals. Some nutrient functions certainly are known, thanks to exhaustive clinical research and empirical data. However, there are many functions that *seem* to be known, and many instances in which nutrients interrelate with each other to such a degree that one cannot clearly differentiate the activity of one from another. Known functions, then, are those ways in which nutrients are thought to participate in regular body functions. Vitamin A, for example, promotes growth and vitality. So do several other vitamins. A flexible approach to the known functions categories will give you a better feel for the fluid, interrelatedness of nutrition, and for the activity of vitamins and minerals.

Solubility: This category is applicable to vitamins only, and has to do with their ability to be absorbed within the gastrointestinal tract. Vitamins must dissolve into solution before they can be absorbed and utilized by the body. Water soluble vitamins are those which can dissolve in water, or in the natural, waterbased fluids which keep the digestive tract moist. Oil soluble vitamins are those which do not dissolve in water, but instead require an oily medium or an emulsifier such as bile, which is manufactured by the liver, to break down the vitamins into assimilable particles.

Insufficiency Signs: As with the category of known functions, this category also lacks the certainty of mathematical precision. Insufficiency signs are those ways by which the body expresses the complex problems of an inadequate dietary intake of any or all nutrients. For example, bleeding gums are typical of a vitamin C insufficiency. However, there are so many indicators, both gross and subtle, attributable to inadequate nutrition, that the proper identification of a particular nutrient insufficiency is often quite impossible. Lack of vigor, poor growth, and chronic fatigue can be indicative of any number of several nutrient insufficiencies. Thus many indicators must be regarded as expressions of an "insufficiency complex," the result of several imbalances in the body, most likely caused by the inadequate dietary intake of more than just one, single nutrient. More often than not, this is in fact the case.

RDA: This category lists the current Recommended Dietary Allowances for the twelve essential vitamins and the seven essential minerals officially recognized by the United States Food and Drug Administration. Separate listings are given for:

Children twelve months to four years of age
Adults and children four years or older
Pregnant or lactating women

Antagonize or Deplete: This category lists for each nutrient those substances known or suspected to destroy, inhibit, deplete, or otherwise interfere with the activity of that nutrient. In some cases the antagonism or depletion is not only known, but the exact mechanism for it is understood. In other cases, the antagonism or depletion is known, but the mechanism is not understood. And in yet other cases, the antagonism or depletion is suspected but not yet confirmed.

Nutrient Measure and Conversion Chart

	Weights	
1 kilogram	=	1,000 grams
1 gram	=	1,000 milligrams (mg.)
1 milligram	=	1/1,000th of a gram
1 microgram	=	1/1,000th of a milligram
28.35 grams	=	1 ounce
454 grams	=	1 pound
1 grain	=	0.0648 grams, or
	=	65 milligrams
	Liquids	
1 minim*	=	0.0038 cubic inches
60 minims	=	1 fluid dram
8 fluid drams	=	1 fluid ounce

*A *minim* is measure of liquid volume, and therefore is not convertible to milligram value, as a milligram is a measure of weight.

124/VITAMINS, MINERALS, AND FOOD SUPPLEMENTS

Vitamin E used to be measured in milligrams, but is now measured in International Units. The following I.U. values per milligram of four different forms of E indicate varying degrees of activity.

1 unit of E activity=1 milligram dl-alpha tocopherol acetate.
1 mg. dl-alpha tocopherol=1.1 International Units.
1 mg. d-alpha tocopheryl acetate=1.36 I.U.
1 mg. d-alpha tocopherol=1.49 I.U.
1 mg. d-alpha tocopheryl acid succinate=1.21 I.U.

For Vitamin A and Beta-Carotene,

1 I.U. Vitamin A=0.3 mcg. A alcohol
3,300 I.U. Vitamin A=1 mg. A alcohol
1 I.U. Vitamin A=0.6 mcg. Beta-Carotene
1 11,000 I.U. capsule of Beta-Carotene=6.6 mg. Beta-Carotene

Vitamins:	*Minerals:*
A (Retinol)	Calcium
B_1 (Thiamine)	Magnesium
B_2 (Riboflavin)	Phosphorous
Niacin	Iodine
B_6 (Pyridoxine)	Iron
B_{12} (Cyanocobalamin)	Copper
Pantothenic Acid	Zinc
PABA (Para-Amino-Benzoic-Acid)*	Sodium**
Folic Acid (Folacin)	Potassium**
Biotin	Manganese**
Choline*	Selenium**
Inositol*	Chromium**
Vitamin C (Ascorbic Acid)	
Vitamin D	
Vitamin E	
"Vitamin F" (Essential Fatty Acids)*	
Vitamin K (Phylloquinone)	
Vitamin P (Bioflavonoids)*	

*Not officially recognized by the U.S. FDA as a vitamin.
**U.S.—RDA has not been established.

Vitamin A (Retinol)

Sources: Eggs, liver, kidney, fish liver oil, fish, dark green and yellow vegetables, milk, dairy products, butter, hot red peppers, peaches, cantaloupe.

Known Functions: Builds resistance to infection. Promotes growth and vitality. Necessary for pregnancy and lactation. Forms rhodopsin (otherwise known as visual purple), which is necessary for good vision and night sight. Helps growth, maintenance and repair of healthy skin and lining tissues, hair, teeth, bones, and glands.

Solubility: Fat soluble.

Insufficiency Signs: Night blindness, tooth or gum decay, dry or scaly skin, acne, loss of appetite, stunted growth, loss of vigor, sinus trouble, increased susceptibility to infection, eye irritations.

RDA: Children twelve months to four years of age—2,500 I.U.
Adults and children four years or older—5,000 I.U.
Pregnant or lactating women—8,000 I.U.

Antagonize or Deplete: Caffeine, mineral oil, excessive iron, vitamin D deficiency, cholesteramine, neomycin.

Vitamin B_1 (Thiamine)

Sources: Rice bran, sunflower seeds, nuts, egg yolks, poultry, pork, beef, lamb, organ meats, fish, dried peas and beans, brown rice, legumes, whole wheat, blackstrap molasses, brewer's yeast.

Known Functions: Promotes growth. Maintenance of healthy nervous system, particularly peripheral nerve tissue. Needed for function of heart, muscle coordination, digestion, proper intestinal muscle tone, learning capacity, and metabolism of carbohydrates.

Solubility: Water soluble.

Insufficiency Signs: Loss of appetite, mental depression, irritability, weight loss, constipation, insomnia, shortness of breath, impaired growth in children, weakness, fatigue, nervousness, cramping and numbness in legs, vague aches and pains, neuritis, beriberi.

RDA: Children twelve months to four years of age—0.7 mg.
Adults and children four years or older—1.5 mg.
Pregnant or lactating women—1.7 mg.

Antagonize or Deplete: Caffeine, tobacco, alcohol, stress, fever.

Vitamin B₂ (Riboflavin)

Sources: Egg yolks, milk, cheese, brewer's yeast, blackstrap molasses, wheat germ, organ meats, whole grains, green leafy vegetables.

Known Functions: Promotes healthy eyes, skin and mouth. Functions in the conversion of fats and carbohydrates into useable energy. Necessary for red blood and antibody formation.

Solubility: Water soluble.

Insufficiency Signs: Cracking of lips and corners of the mouth, bloodshot eyes, itching and burning of the eyes, inflammation of mouth, swollen and purple tongue, dizziness, poor digestion.

RDA: Children twelve months to four years of age—0.8 mg.
Adults and children four years or older—1.7 mg.
Pregnant or lactating women—2.0 mg.

Antagonize or Deplete: Alcohol, sugar, caffeine, tobacco.

Niacin

Sources: Green vegetables, nuts, lean meats, milk, rice bran, brewer's yeast, beans, poultry, fish, desiccated liver, whole grains.

Known Functions: Metabolism of carbohydrates, fats, and proteins, and normal function of gastrointestinal tract. Needed for healthy skin, mouth and nervous system. Dilates blood vessels and improves circulation.

Solubility: Water soluble.

Insufficiency Signs: Pellagra (the symptoms of which include inflammation of the skin and tongue), headaches, mental depression, fatigue, irritability, weakness, weight loss, insomnia, vague aches and pains, gastrointestinal disturbances, loss of appetite, neuritis.

RDA: Children twelve months to four years of age—9 mg.
Adults and children four years or older—20 mg.
Pregnant or lactating women—20 mg.

Antagonize or Deplete: Sugar, caffeine, alcohol, antibiotics, isoniazid.

Vitamin B₆ (Pyridoxine)

Sources: Meat, fish, wheat germ, egg yolk, cantaloupe, avocado, bananas, cabbage, grapes, carrots, peas, potatoes, leafy greens, milk, legumes, brewer's yeast, blackstrap molasses, walnuts, peanuts, prunes.

Known Functions: Aids food assimilation, protein and fat metabolism, use of amino acids in the body, and formation of certain proteins. Important for healthy nervous system, digestion, production of red blood cells, weight control.

Solubility: Water soluble.

Insufficiency Signs: Nervousness, loss of muscle control, skin eruptions, insomnia, anemia, irritability, depression, hair loss, insulin sensitivity, learning disabilities.

RDA: Children twelve months to four years of age—0.7 mg.
      Adults and children four years or older—2.0 mg.
      Pregnant or lactating women—2.5 mg.

Antagonize or Deplete: Alcohol, caffeine, tobacco, radiation exposure, estrogen-containing contraceptives, hydralazine, isoniazid, penicillamine.

Vitamin B₁₂ (Cyanocobalamin)

Sources: Liver, beef, pork, eggs, milk, cheese, shellfish, sardines, salmon, herring, organ meats, pollen.

Known Functions: Essential to the synthesis of hemoglobin, construction and regeneration of red blood cells. Antianemia factor, metabolism of all foods, healthy nervous system, normal appetite, promotes growth and appetite in children. General tonic for adults. Antidepressive in large doses.

Solubility: Water soluble.

Insufficiency Signs: Fatigue, general weakness, loss of appetite, anemia, neuritis, poor growth in children.

RDA: Children twelve months to four years of age—3 mcg.
      Adults and children four years or older—6 mcg.
      Pregnant or lactating women—8 mcg.

Antagonize or Deplete: Tobacco, caffeine, alcohol, most laxatives, cholesteramine,

128/Vitamins, Minerals, and Food Supplements

colchicine, estrogen-containing oral contraceptives, neomycin, para-amino-salicylic acid, potassium chloride.

Pantothenic Acid

Sources: Liver, egg yolks, kidney, salmon, brewer's yeast, whole grains, soybeans, wheat germ, bran, green vegetables, legumes, blackstrap molasses.

Known Functions: Essential for the formation of various regulating substances and hormones, for digestion of carbohydrates, proteins, and fats, and for utilization of vitamins. Involved in building of body cells, normal skin, digestive function, resistance to stress, formation of antibodies, health of adrenal glands.

Solubility: Water soluble.

Insufficiency Signs: Retarded growth, burning feet, dizziness, hypoglycemia, allergies, digestive troubles, chronic fatigue, skin disorders.

RDA: Children twelve months to four years of age—5 mg.
Adults and children four years or older—10 mg.
Pregnant or lactating women—10 mg.

Antagonize or Deplete: Alcohol, sugar, caffeine.

PABA (Para-Amino-Benzoic Acid)

Sources: Wheat germ, brewer's yeast, yogurt, milk, eggs, organ meats, rice bran, blackstrap molasses, leafy green vegetables.

Known Functions: Growth promoting factor, red blood cell formation, health of skin, natural sunscreen, maintenance of skin pigmentation and hair color, promotes healthy intestinal flora, assists in protein metabolism.

Solubility: Water soluble.

Insufficiency Signs: Anemia, eczema, extreme fatigue, loss of hair color and skin pigmentation, constipation, headaches, nervousness.

RDA: No U.S.—RDA has been established.

Antagonize or Deplete: Caffeine, alcohol, sulfonamides.

Folic Acid (Folacin)

Sources: Leafy greens, wheat germ, bran, broccoli, brewer's yeast, nuts, whole grains, milk products, beans, organ meats, oysters, tuna.

Known Functions: Formation of red blood cells, formation of various body proteins and genetic materials for the cell nucleus. Involved in reproduction and growth, healthy glands and liver, healthy hair. Contributes to normal growth, assists protein metabolism, aids in prevention of macrocytic anemia.

Solubility: Water soluble.

Insufficiency Signs: Macrocytic anemia, reproductive disorders, loss of libido in males, retarded growth, graying and loss of hair, gastrointestinal disorders.

RDA: Children twelve months to four years of age—0.2 mg.
Adults and children four years or older—0.4 mg.
Pregnant or lactating women—0.8 mg.

Antagonize or Deplete: Stress, alcohol, caffeine, tobacco, anticonvulsants, cholesteramine, estrogen-containing oral contraceptives, methotrexate, pryimethamine, salicylates, sulphasalizine, triamterene, trimethoprim.

Biotin

Sources: Whole grains, egg yolks, legumes, chicken, liver, kidney, sardines, nuts, brewer's yeast.

Known Functions: Healthy skin, hair, and muscles, metabolism of carbohydrates, proteins, fats. Assists utilization of folic acid, pantothenic acid, niacin. Involved in body growth, fatty acid production, maintenance of thyroid, adrenal glands, nervous system, reproductive system.

Solubility: Water soluble.

Insufficiency Signs: Exhaustion, drowsiness, loss of appetite, mental depression, anemia, skin disorders, muscle pain, hair loss.

RDA: Children twelve months to four years of age—0.15 mg.
Adults and children four years or older—0.3 mg.
Pregnant or lactating women—0.3 mg.

Antagonize or Deplete: Alcohol, avidin (found in raw egg whites).

Choline

Sources: Lecithin, wheat germ, whole grains, legumes, soybeans, fish, egg yolks, organ meats, leafy green vegetables, brewer's yeast.

Known Functions: Fat metabolism, normal nerve transmission, health of the liver, brain and memory functions.

Solubility: Water soluble.

Insufficiency Signs: Fatty liver, hardening of the arteries, intolerance to fats, high blood pressure, impaired memory.

RDA: No U.S.—RDA has been established.

Antagonize or Deplete: Alcohol.

Inositol

Sources: Fruits, nuts, wheat germ, whole grains, milk, meat, brewer's yeast.

Known Functions: Metabolism of fats and cholesterol, health of liver.

Solubility: Water soluble.

Insufficiency Signs: Poor metabolism of fats, high cholesterol levels.

RDA: No U.S.—RDA has been established.

Antagonize or Deplete: Alcohol.

Vitamin C (Ascorbic Acid)

Sources: Citrus fruits, tomatoes, green peppers, strawberries, kale, parsley, alfalfa sprouts, papaya, broccoli, hot red peppers, cabbage, cauliflower.

Known Functions: Aids in production of collagen, which gives structure to muscles, vascular tissues, bones and cartilage. Contributes to healthy teeth and gums. Aids iron absorbtion, promotes wound healing, general immunity. Maintains capillary integrity, assists in production of interferon. Antioxidant.

Solubility: Water soluble.

Insufficiency Signs: Scurvy, soft gums, tooth decay, loss of appetite, muscular weakness, skin hemorrhages, anemia, increased susceptibility to colds and flu, capillary fragility, overall diminished immunity.

RDA: Children twelve months to four years of age—40 mg.
Adults and children four years or older—60 mg.
Pregnant or lactating women—60 mg.

Antagonize or Deplete: Stress, fever, alcohol, caffeine, tobacco, pollution, estrogen-containing oral contraceptives, salicylates, tetracycline.

Vitamin D

Sources: Fish liver oils, grain and vegetable oils, butter, exposure to the sun, sardines, salmon, tuna, mushrooms.

Known Functions: Utilization of calcium and phosphorous, proper formation of bones and teeth, healthy skin.

Solubility: Oil soluble.

Insufficiency Signs: Rickets, tooth decay, lack of vigor, stunted growth, porous bones, diarrhea, nervousness, muscular weakness.

RDA: Children twelve months to four years of age—400 I.U.
Adults and children four years or older—400 I.U.
Pregnant or lactating women—400 I.U.

Antagonize or Deplete: Mineral oil, anticonvulsants, cholesteramine, glutethimide, irritant cathartics.

Vitamin E

Sources: Wheat germ, nuts, nut and seed oils, eggs, organ meats, oatmeal, olives.

Known Functions: Helps prevent sterility, improves circulation, promotes longevity, prevents blood clots, prolongs life of red blood cells, strengthens capillary walls, helps body utilize vitamin A, maintains integrity of cell membranes. Antioxidant, antiabortive. Contributes to healthy skin, hair.

Solubility: Oil soluble.

Insufficiency Signs: Increased fragility of red blood cells, varicose veins, sterility, cystic mastitis, spontaneous abortion, heart disease, stroke.

RDA: Children twelve months to four years of age—10 I.U.
Adults and children four years or older—30 I.U.
Pregnant or lactating women—30 I.U.

Antagonize or Deplete: Mineral oil, rancid fats and oils.

"Vitamin F" (Unsaturated Fatty Acids)

Sources: Vegetable oils such as soybean, peanut, sesame, safflower, cottonseed, corn and linseed, butter, nuts and seeds, wheat germ.

Known Functions: Promotes growth, healthy hair and skin, normal glandular activity, regulation of cholesterol, body lubrication and resilience, availability of calcium to the cells, healthy arteries.

Solubility: Oil soluble.

Insufficiency Signs: Acne, dandruff, dry hair, diarrhea, weak nails, arthritis, menstrual disorders.

RDA: No. U.S.—RDA has been established.

Antagonize or Deplete: Mineral oil.

Vitamin K (Phylloquinone)

Sources: Alfalfa, leafy green vegetables, cauliflower, kelp, soybeans, soybean oil, egg yolks.

Known Functions: Assists production of prothrombin, which is essential to proper clotting of the blood. Important to healthy liver function.

Solubility: Oil soluble.

Insufficiency Signs: Hemorrhages resulting from slow clotting time, nosebleeds.

RDA: No U.S.—RDA has been established.

Antagonize or Deplete: Mineral oil, antibiotics, sulfa drugs.

The Nutrient Section/133

Vitamin P (Bioflavonoids, including citrus bioflavonoids, rutin, hesperidin)

Sources: Peels and pulp of citrus fruits, buckwheat, black currants, cherries, grapes, bell peppers.

Known Functions: Believed to strengthen capillary walls, protect vitamin C from being destroyed in the body by oxidation, aid resistance to colds and flu, prevent bruising, aids hypertension.

Solubility: Water soluble.

Insufficiency signs: Bruising, increased susceptibility to colds and flu, varicose veins, capillary fragility, with appearance of purplish spots on the skin.

RDA: No U.S.—RDA has been established.

Antagonize or Deplete: Excessive copper or iron.

Calcium

Sources: Milk, cheese, yogurt, bone meal, dolomite, shellfish, salmon, sardines, almonds, sesame seeds, liver, leafy green vegetables, blackstrap molasses.

Known Functions: Growth and maintenance of teeth and bones, blood clotting, nerve transmission and tranquilization, heart rhythm, vitality and endurance, muscle growth.

Insufficiency Signs: Stunted growth, rickets, nerve disorders, fragile or porous bones, tooth decay, menstrual cramps, heart palpitations, foot and leg cramps.

RDA: Children twelve months to four years of age—0.8 gm. (800 mg.)
Adults and children four years or older—1 gm. (1,000 mg.)
Pregnant or lactating women—1.3 gm. (1,300 mg.)

Antagonize or Deplete: Stress, excess or lack of magnesim, lack of hydrochloric acid, excessive intake of oxalic acid (which occurs in spinach, rhubarb and cranberries), phytic acid (which occurs in soybeans), excess phosphorous.

Magnesium

Sources: Dairy products (except butter), whole grains, dried beans and peas, soybeans, nuts, leafy green vegetables, dolomite, wheat germ, bran.

Known Functions: Essential to all living cells and to utilization of calcium. Catalyst in many biological reactions, needed for nerve transmission, muscle contractions, healthy bones, arteries, heart, teeth.

Insufficiency Signs: Poor utilization of calcium, tremors, nervousness, irritability, constipation.

RDA: Children twelve months or four years of age—200 mg.
Adults and children four years or older—400 mg.
Pregnant or lactating women—450 mg.

Antagonize or Deplete: Excess calcium or phosphorous.

Phosphorous

Sources: Eggs, fish, grains, organ meats, poultry, meat, cheese, nuts and seeds, legumes, milk, bran, wheat germ, lecithin, yeast.

Known Functions: Proper growth of bones and teeth, growth and repair of cells, nerve and muscle activity, carbohydrate metabolism, heart muscle contraction, balancing of pH levels in the body.

Insufficiency Signs: Weakness, poor formation of bones and teeth, nervous disorders, loss of appetite, fatigue, impaired calcium absorption.

RDA: Children twelve months to four years of age—0.8 gm. (800 mg.)
Adults and children four years or older—1 gm. (1,000 mg.)
Pregnant or lactating women—1.3 gm. (1,300 mg.)

Antagonize or Deplete: Sugar, excessive intakes of magnesium, aluminum, iron, calcium.

Iodine

Sources: Seafood, kelp, dulse, chard, garlic, Irish moss, mushrooms.

Known Functions: Healthy thyroid, regulation of metabolism, energy production, healthy hair, skin, nails, teeth.

Insufficiency Signs: Thyroid disorders, obesity, goiter, irritability, nervousness, dry hair, cold hands and feet.

RDA: Children twelve months to four years of age—70 mcg.
   Adults and children four years or older—150 mcg.
   Pregnant or lactating women—150 mcg.

Antagonize or Deplete: Brassica plants, including cabbage, turnip, mustard, and related species.

Iron

Sources: Liver, eggs, fish, poultry, kelp, rice bran, blackstrap molasses, apricots, raisins, wheat germ, sunflower seeds, parsley.

Known Functions: Manufacture of hemoglobin, oxygen transport in the blood, resistance to disease, improved energy, healthy teeth, skin, nails and bones.

Insufficiency Signs: Fatigue, anemia, paleness, brittle nails, constipation, difficulty in breathing.

RDA: Children twelve months to four years of age—10 mg.
   Adults and children four years or older—18 mg.
   Pregnant or lactating women—18 mg.

Antagonize or Deplete: Caffeine, excessive phosphorous, zinc, or copper.

Copper

Sources: Whole grains, seafood, organ meats, mushrooms, raisins, nuts, legumes, blackstrap molasses.

Known Functions: Bone formation, red blood cell production, hair and skin color.

Insufficiency Signs: Weakness, anemia, hair loss, poor respiration, retarded growth.

RDA: Children twelve months to four years of age—1 mg.
   Adults and children four years or older—2 mg.
   Pregnant or lactating women—2 mg.

Antagonize or Deplete: Excessive zinc.

Zinc

Sources: Milk, eggs, seafood, liver, oysters, mushrooms, wheat germ, bran, nuts, leafy greens.

Known Functions: Protein and carbohydrate metabolism, prostate gland function, healthy reproductive organs, bone formation, wound and burn healing.

Insufficiency Signs: Fatigue, hair loss, enlarged prostate, delayed sexual maturity, diminished libido, poor wound healing, sterility.

RDA: Children twelve months to four years of age—8 mg.
Adults and children four years or older—15 mg.
Pregnant or lactating women—15 mg.

Antagonize or Deplete: Alcohol, phosphorous deficiency, excessive calcium, copper, or iron.

Sodium

Sources: Salt, seafood, kelp, dulse, poultry, meat, cheese, green olives.

Known Functions: Works with potassium to equalize acid-alkaline balance of blood, helps regulate balance of water in body. Involved in muscle contractions.

Insufficiency Signs: Dehydration, poor muscle function, blood pH imbalance.

RDA: No U.S.—RDA has been established.

Antagonize or Deplete: Excessive sweating, diuretics, extreme dieting, excess potassium.

Potassium

Sources: Leafy greens, bananas, seafood, apricots, figs, raisins, parsley, kelp, wheat germ, blackstrap molasses, potato.

Known Functions: Normal growth, muscle contraction, proper alkalinity of body fluids, regular heartbeat, proper nerve function, kidney function, works with sodium to maintain water balance in body.

Insufficiency Signs: General weakness, nervousness, constipation, dry skin, tendency toward muscle damage, cardiac arrest, insomnia, acne.

RDA: No U.S.—RDA has been established.

Antagonize or Deplete: Sugar, caffeine, most diuretics, alcohol, stress, excess sodium, most laxatives, cortisone.

Manganese

Sources: Leafy green vegetables, parsley, carrots, celery, beets, wheat germ, bran, nuts, whole grains, meat.

Known Functions: Digestion of fats, reproduction and growth, sex hormone production, enzyme activation.

Insufficiency Signs: Stunted growth, sterility, loss of hearing, dizziness.

RDA: No U.S.—RDA has been established.

Antagonize or Deplete: Excessive intake of phosphorous, calcium, or iron.

Selenium

Sources: Eggs, milk, mushrooms, brewer's yeast, whole grains, tuna, wheat bran, wheat germ, onions, broccoli.

Known Functions: Antioxidant, assists vitamin E, preserves tissue elasticity, promotes healthy function of testicles, believed to enhance immunity to carcinogens, or possibly inhibit tumor or cancer growth.

Insufficiency Signs: Premature aging, impaired male sexual function, dandruff, possible enhanced predisposition to cancer and tumors.

RDA: No U.S.—RDA has been established.

Antagonize or Deplete: None known.

Chromium

Sources: Whole grains, brewer's yeast, clams, corn oil.

138/Vitamins, Minerals, and Food Supplements

Known Functions: Assists glucose tolerance, healthy blood circulation, production of insulin and increased insulin effectiveness, synthesis of fatty acids, cholesterol and protein.

Insufficiency Signs: Depressed growth rate, hypoglycemia, arteriosclerosis.

RDA: No U.S.—RDA has been established.

Antagonize or Deplete: None known.

Nature—Vite Quick Reference Chart

A list of vitamins and minerals, and several sources from which they are obtained.

Vitamin A: Fish liver oil, liver, milk, hot red peppers, dandelion greens, carrots, apricots, kale, leafy greens, fertile eggs, yellow dock, lamb's quarters.

Vitamin C: Acerola cherries, hot red peppers, parsley, black currants, kale, all citrus fruits, rose hips, strawberries, green peppers.

Vitamin D: Sunlight, fish liver oil, salmon, sardines, tuna, milk, eggs, mushrooms.

Vitamin E: Wheat germ, rice germ, brown rice, nuts, eggs, leafy greens, nut and seed oils, olive oil, oats, liver, organ meats.

"Vitamin F" (unsaturated fatty acids): Nuts, seeds, nut and seed oils, olives, corn, avocados, wheat germ.

Vitamin K: Greens, alfalfa, kelp, eggs, cauliflower, soybeans, soy oil, yogurt, blackstrap molasses, fish liver oil.

Vitamin B_1 (thiamine): Rice bran, sunflower seeds, wheat germ, nuts and seeds, brewer's yeast, egg yolks, poultry, pork, beef, lamb, organ meats, fish.

Vitamin B_2 (riboflavin): Hot red peppers, almonds, wheat germ, sunflower seeds, milk, cheese, brewer's yeast, egg yolks, organ meats.

Vitamin B_3 (niacin): Rice bran, rice polish, torula yeast, wheat bran, brewer's yeast, green vegetables, lean meats, poultry, fish.

Vitamin B_6 (pyridoxine): Brewer's yeast, avocados, blackstrap molasses, bananas, wheat germ, wheat bran, egg yolks, leafy greens, meat, fish.

PABA: Rice polish, rice bran, wheat germ, brewer's yeast, yogurt, milk, eggs, organ meats.

Biotin: Brewer's yeast, nuts, whole grains, chicken, liver, kidney, sardines.

Folic Acid: Mushrooms, leafy greens, soybeans, wheat germ, broccoli, brewer's yeast, nuts, milk products, organ meats, oysters, tuna.

Pantothenic Acid: Rice polish, soybeans, wheat germ, whole grains, green vegetables, liver, egg yolks, kidney, salmon, legumes, blackstrap molasses.

Lecithin: Soybeans, egg yolks.

Choline: Soybeans, turnips, leafy greens, wheat germ, nuts, lecithin, brewer's yeast, fish, egg yolks, organ meats.

Inositol: Grapefruit, orange, wheat germ, nuts, whole grains, brewer's yeast, milk, meat.

Vitamin B_{12} (cyanocobalamin): Comfrey, spirulina, kelp, eggs, milk, wheat germ, pollen, cheese, fish, liver, beef, pork, shellfish, sardines, salmon, herring, organ meats.

Orotic Acid: Whey.

Bioflavonoids, Rutin, Hesperidin: Buckwheat, black currants, cherries, grapes, citrus fruits, green peppers.

Calcium: Sesame seed, kelp, Irish moss, agar, dulse, lamb's quarters, blackstrap molasses, milk, cheese, bone meal, shellfish, salmon, sardines, leafy green vegetables.

Potassium: Dulse, kelp, Irish moss, leafy greens, bananas, blackstrap molasses, apricots, figs, parsley, wheat germ, raisins, potatoes, seafood.

Magnesium: Kelp, wheat bran, wheat germ, almonds, sesame, leafy greens, cashews, soybeans, Brazil nuts, dairy products.

Iron: Dulse, kelp, rice bran, blackstrap molasses, apricots, raisins, wheat germ, sunflower seeds, parsley, liver, eggs, fish, poultry.

Phosphorous: Rice bran, wheat bran, pumpkin seeds, wheat germ, nuts, seeds, eggs, fish, meat, poultry, cheese.

Iodine: Kelp, dulse, agar, Swiss chard, garlic, Irish moss, seafood.

Manganese: Parsley, carrots, celery, beets, leafy greens, wheat germ, wheat bran, nuts, whole grains, meat.

Zinc: Wheat germ, eggs, milk, brewer's yeast, bran, nuts, leafy greens, seafood, liver, oysters.

Sodium: Salt, kelp, Irish moss, dulse, olives, celery, watermelon, blackstrap molasses, meat, cheese.

Sulfur: Kale, watercress, Brussels sprouts, horseradish, soybeans, dried beans, peanuts, oats.

Copper: Currants, mushrooms, raisins, nuts, legumes, whole grains, leafy greens, seafood, organ meats.

Chlorine: Tomatoes, celery, iceberg lettuce, kelp, oats, parsley, blackstrap molasses, bananas, coconut, kale.

Selenium: Brewer's yeast, eggs, milk, mushrooms, tuna.

Silicon: Lettuce, parsnips, asparagus, strawberries, cucumbers, alfalfa.

Fluorine: Almonds, beet greens, carrots, turnip greens, milk, cheese, garlic.

Germanium: Ginseng, garlic, onions.

Chromium: Brewer's yeast, meats, cheese, whole grains.

Molybdenum: Meat, whole grains, legumes.

Food Supplements

The following is a list of items which are used in the same manner as vitamins and minerals, but which are actually food derived or naturally derived. These food supplements are nutritionally concentrated, and have therapeutic value as well.

Acidophilus: Actually a bacteria, lactobacillus acidophilus is found in the intestinal tracts of healthy people, and is active in cleaning up unwanted debris in the gastro-intestinal tract. Acidophilus is typically used as a yogurt culture. Eaten daily, acidophilus enhances digestive and eliminative activity, aids the body's production of B-vitamins, and enhances immunity. The only actual acidophilus products which are viable are those which have been refrigerated. Mega Dophilus is such a brand.

Beta-Carotene: A yellow or red pigment found naturally in colored fruits and vegetables, egg yolk, milk fat, and body fat, beta-carotene is made up of two molecules of vitamin A linked end to end. Enzymes in the human liver split each molecule of beta carotene into two molecules of vitamin A. Beta-carotene performs the same functions as vitamin A, and has been shown to be of value in reducing the risk of a variety of types of cancer.

Bio Strath: This yeast elixir mixed with herbs is used to increase energy, reduce fatigue, and enhance immunity, and is valuable in fighting unwanted strains of bacteria in the body. Bio Strath is heavily researched, and has been proven to improve concentration, and increase stamina and endurance. It is particularly useful for children, as it has a very pleasant taste.

Bone Meal: Made from the dried, ground bones of cattle, bone meal is high in calcium and phosphorous. Bone meal is of value for the growth and maintenance of teeth and bones, blood clotting, nerve transmission, nerve tranquilization, heart rhythm, vitality and endurance, muscle growth, growth and repair of cells, carbohydrate metabolism, and heart muscle contraction.

Desiccated Liver: This is liver that has been dried, and usually defatted as well. Liver is an excellent source of protein, iron, and B-vitamins, and has a long-standing reputation as an energy enhancing food. Desiccated liver is typically used as a protein supplement, and as a concentrated food for athletes. It is also of value to anemics, due to its high concentration of iron and B-vitamins.

Digestants: The process of digestion involves the activity of several enzymes. Enzymes are usually protein-containing compounds which are interconnected with vitamins or minerals in many cases. Digestive enzymes function to reduce foods to their usable components, enabling the body to utilize the foods for fuel, growth and maintenance. With the exception of Betaine HCL, the following substances are all enzymes:

Betaine HCL: In the stomach, hydrochloric acid is secreted both to break down protein foods into simpler components, and to provide an acid climate for pepsin, an "acid loving" enzyme. Secretion of stomach acid can be diminished by poor dietary habits, stress, and old age. Betaine HCL supplements the body's natural stomach acid, enhancing the digestive climate.

Bromelain: Bromelain is a protein digesting enzyme which is found in pineapple. Taken in supplement form, bromelain enhances the digestion of protein. It also acts as an anti-inflammatory agent, and is prescribed therapeutically for pain and inflammation of joints and muscles.

Ox Bile: Bile is a fluid secreted by the liver, and then conveyed to the small intestine. Bile enhances the alkaline climate of the intestine, helps to emulsify fats, and inhibits putrefaction. Bile also lubricates the intestines, thus enhancing bowel activity. Supplementary bile stimulates the secretory activity of the liver, enhancing the liver's own bile production. One of the compounds in bile is cholic acid, which is active in the emulsification, dispersal, and absorption of fats, cholesterol, and oil-soluble vitamins.

Pancreatin: Pancreatin is a complex of digestive factors produced by the pancreas, and used in the small intestine. Pancreatin contains amylase, chymotrypsin, lipase, trypsin.

Amylase: Amylase works only on carbohydrates, breaking down starches into simpler sugars.

Chymotrypsin: This enzyme catalyzes the breakdown of certain amino acids. As such, it is a specific protein-digesting enzyme.

Lipase: This enzyme splits up fats, and is directly connected with the metabolism of fatty acids. It is considered to be the most important fat digesting enzyme in the entire digestive process.

Trypsin: This enzyme is proteolytic, meaning that it breaks down proteins.

Papain: This protein-digesting enzyme is derived from the papaya fruit, and is used both as a supplementary digestant and commercially in meat tenderizing products.

Pepsin: This proteolytic enzyme occurs in the stomach, and as stated before, requires an acidic climate for proper activity. Pepsin starts the process of protein digestion, along with hydrochloric acid.

Dolomite: This is a simple soft stone which contains calcium and magnesium in a balance of 2 to 1 respectively. In the human body, calcium and magnesium are used in this proportion to one another. Dolomite is an excellent, inexpensive way to obtain these two minerals.

Evening Primrose Oil: This oil from the flower of the evening primrose contains GLA (gamma linolenic acid), which is needed for the production of a hormone-like substance known as Prostaglandin E1. This substance is important for the health of the nervous system, immune system, cardiovascular system, reproductive system, skin, and metabolism. Primrose oil is a concentrated source of GLA, which is found in concentration only in mother's milk and spirulina, a micro-algae. The only reliable brand of primrose oil at this time is Efamol.

Kyolic: This is a specially processed garlic product made by Wakunaga, a Japanese pharmaceutical company. It is effective for all of the uses of garlic, including increasing energy and immunity. However, this garlic is very concentrated, and does not have the garlic odor. Thus it is a highly versatile item. *Kyolic* comes in liquid or tablet form; the liquid is more concentrated.

L-lysine: This is an essential amino acid, one of the fundamental building products of protein. It is used by consumers to minimize the incidence of herpes.

L-tryptophan: This is another essential amino acid. It is used as a sleep aid, and is taken (approx. 500 mg.) about twenty minutes prior to retiring.

MaxEPA: MaxEPA is a fish body oil which is high in two particular fatty acids, EPA, and DHA. MaxEPA has been proven to reduce serum LDL cholesterol levels, reduce serum triglyceride levels, and reduce platelet aggregation. More simply stated, MaxEPA cleans the arteries, reducing the risk of heart disease.

Octacosanol: From the oil of the germ of the whole wheat kernel, octacosanol is derived. Octacosanol has been shown to enhance muscle glycogen storage, improve stability of basal metabolic rate under stress, reduce oxygen debt, improve total body reaction capabilities, improve post exercise recovery time, enhance response to stress, increase muscular strength, and improve stamina and endurance.

Propolis: This is a substance made by bees from the sap of trees. Propolis is highly antibacterial and antibiotic, and can be consumed as an alternative to manufactured antibiotic drugs. Propolis is also high in bioflavonoids, which assist the health and integrity of cell membranes. It is commonly used in either tablet or liquid form for colds, flu, and other ailments which involve immune resistance.

Royal Jelly: This is the substance fed to queen bees by their attendants. Royal Jelly is a thick, creamy substance which is loaded with natural hormones. It has been prized for centuries as a vitality elixir, an aphrodisiac, and a rejuvenator.

Spirulina: This is a fresh water micro-algae which is high in protein, vitamins, chlorophyll, and GLA, the same fatty acid described earlier under the heading of evening primrose oil. Spirulina is used as a protein supplement, it is taken by athletes for extra energy, and it is used as a supplement during fasting, as it is easily digested.

Zell Oxygen: This is the live, liquid counterpart to brewer's yeast. Zell Oxygen is teeming with live yeast cells which have been saturated with oxygen by a special process. It is useful in instances of breathing difficulties, sleeplessness, chronic fatigue, weakness, and sexual debility. It is expensive, but entirely worth the price.

HERBOLOGY

Herbs, What They Are, What They Do

Herbs are a group of botanical substances which have been used therapeutically for thousands of years by every group of people in every nation. They have been the foundation of the materia medica of all traditional health care systems. In fact, until just the last one hundred years, herbs were used in almost all instances in which medication was required for the treatment of illness. Generation after generation of successful herbalists have tested and refined the vast science of herbology, so that today it is one of the most complete, sophisticated, and effective of all health care systems. The proper and judicious use of herbs has been successful in the treatment of illness when other, more orthodox methods of treatment have failed. Herbs are generally safe, natural, and used as nature grew them. Unlike dangerous pharmaceutical drugs, the potency of herbs is in harmony with the natural balance of the environment, and of the human body. Where drugs are often extremely unpredictable in their effects, herbs are more predictable. Where drugs can have lethal side effects, herbs are much safer.

Herbs assist the body's own ability to heal itself. Herbs can be used to cleanse the body, to rebuild tissue, mend broken bones, to purify the blood, stimulate the brain, increase sexual energy, ease pain, aid digestion, and a thousand other purposes. Herbal remedies are currently returning to prominence as effective alternatives to drugs. Botanical medicine is reestablishing itself in the treatment of arthritis, cancer, and other "incurable" illnesses. Thus more high quality herbs are available to the general public than have been for several decades. Most natural food stores have fine selections of teas, loose herbs, and prepared herbal formulas which are ready to use. This is helping to put personal health care back into the hands of the general public, where it should be.

Those who wish to delve into herbology more deeply may enjoy reading *Culpeper's Herbal, The Herbalist*, by Joseph E. Meyer, *School of Natural Healing*, by Dr. John R. Christopher, *Back to Eden*, by Jethro Kloss, and *The Herb Book*, by John Lust. These books will provide the casual reader or the serious student with extensive and enjoyable information.

Preparation and Use of Herbs

Herbal recommendations are given in this book for a variety of ailments and health needs. Herbs suggested are of two categories, herb teas, and prepared herbal formulas.

When *herb teas* are indicated, follow this procedure:

- Boil some water in a stainless steel, enamel, glass, or porcelain pot or pan. Never use aluminum cookware for anything, as it is highly toxic.
- After the water has been brought to a boil, take it off the flame, and pour it

into a pot containing the herbs you are using. These may be either loose herbs, or prepared tea bag formulas. If you are using loose herbs, the ratio of water to herbs is about eight ounces of water to every teaspoon or so of dried herbs. Do not boil the herbs!
- Cover the pot, and let the herbs steep for about five minutes.
- Then strain the tea—do not leave the herbs in the water.
- Let the tea cool a little, and then it is ready to drink.
- You may drink several cups of herb tea daily.

When *prepared herbal formulas* are indicated, follow the directions for use given in this book, or the directions for use appearing on product labels. The prepared herbal formulas recommended in this book are all available at natural food stores.

Individual Herb Chart

The following is a list of some of the most popular common herbs, their botanical names, and a partial list of their medicinal uses. You can use this list as a reference for single medicinal herbs as needed.

Agrimony (*Agrimonia eupatoria*): Fortifies the liver, useful for complaints of the gallbladder, spleen, and kidneys, and for constipation.

Alfalfa (*Medicago sativa*): Digestant that aids in urinary problems. It is high in minerals.

Barberry (*Berberis vulgaris*): Useful in treating all liver complaints, gallbladder problems, chronic bowel troubles, gum disease, diabetes, and poor digestion.

Bayberry (*Myrica cerfera*): Useful in treating hemorrhages, sore throat, diarrhea, dysentery, poor digestion, tonsillitis, and scalp problems. Liver cleanser and glandular stimulant.

Black Cohosh (*Cimicifuga racemosa*): General nerve sedative and cardiac stimulant used to treat bronchitis, rheumatism, arthritis, ulcers, asthma, uterine problems, and seizure disorders.

Blue Cohosh (*Caulophyllum thalictroides*): Menstrual regulator used to treat vaginitis, cramps, exhaustion, diabetes, and high blood pressure. Assists labor.

Buchu (*Barosma crenata*): Diuretic used to treat intestinal gas and bladder and urinary disorders. Induces sweating.

Burdock Root (*Articum lappa*): Blood purifier used for all skin eruptions and inflammation, bladder and kidney disorders, and colds.

Catnip (*Nepeta cataria*): Relaxant and sedative for aches, pains, and nervousness.

Cayenne (*Capsicum annum*): Stimulant that improves circulation, stimulates appetite, and strengthens the digestive system. Decongestant; eliminates mucus. Used for heart trouble, blood pressure problems, colds, constipation, and bleeding. Assists the action of other herbs.

Chamomile (*Anthemis nobelis, Matricaria chamomilla*): Gentle relaxant, soothes stomach, alleviates colic, stomach cramps, and insomnia.

Chaparral (*Larrea tridentata*): Blood cleanser used for stomach disorders, poor digestion, bowel problems, arthritis, cancer, tumors, bladder disorders, skin eruptions, and kidney troubles.

Chia Seed (*Salvia polystachya*): Traditionally used for energy, endurance, and stamina.

Chickweed (*Stellaria media*): Used for all types of tissue and membrane inflammation, bronchitis, asthma, coughs, colds, constipation, tumors, and cancer.

Coltsfoot (*Tussilago farfara*): Useful in treating coughs, colds, bronchitis, asthma, shortness of breath, and hoarseness.

Comfrey Leaf and Root (*Symphytum officinale*): Used for skin problems of any kind, wounds, burns, broken bones, fractures, torn muscles or ligaments, coughs, colds, respiratory difficulties, intestinal mucus, diarrhea, anemia, ulcers, and digestive troubles.

Crampbark (*Viburnum opulus*): Used to treat menstrual cramps, uterine spasms, and nervous disorders.

Damiana (*Turnera aphrodisiaca*): A sexual stimulant and laxative.

Dandelion (*Taraxacum dens-lionis*): Used for liver problems, edema, gallstones, and jaundice; also a detoxifier.

Devil's Claw (*Harpagophytum procumbens*): Used to treat arthritis, rheumatism, inflammations, and swelling.

Echinacea (*Echinacea augustifolia*): Blood purifier, antiseptic, digestant, and aphrodisiac. Used for inflammations, prostate disorders, and bad breath.

Elder (*Sambucus nigra*): Diuretic used for constipation, edema, and kidney problems.

Elecampane (*Inula helenium*): Used for asthma, bronchitis, coughs, digestion, liver trouble, kidney problems, skin eruptions and irritations, and all respiratory ailments. Decongestant; stimulates digestion.

Eucalyptus (*Eucalyptus globulus*): Useful in treating colds, asthma, congestion, and indigestion.

Eyebright (*Euphrasia officinalis*): Used to treat cataracts and other eye ailments.

Fennel (*Feniculum vulgare*): Used for colic, intestinal gas, stomach cramps, and as a diuretic.

Fenugreek (*Trigonella foenum-graecum*): Strengthens the liver; used for sore throat, bronchitis, fevers, and tuberculosis.

Flaxseed (*Linum usitatissimum*): Useful in treating coughs, lung problems, digestive complaints, constipation, and gallstones.

Garlic (*Allium sativum*): Antibacterial, antibiotic, blood purifier, aphrodisiac. Used to treat all respiratory problems, blood-pressure disorders, poor digestion, intestinal gas, skin diseases, tumors, kidney trouble, liver trouble, bladder trouble, colds, flu, and cancer.

Ginger (*Zingiber officinale*): Stimulates appetite and promotes perspiration. Used for colds, flu, coughs, and colic.

Ginseng (*Panax quinquefolius*): Good for everything; general immunity factor, constitutional strengthener, aphrodisiac. Increases energy, stamina, and endurance.

Goldenrod (*Solidago odora*): Used for kidney problems, kidney stones, bladder stones, diarrhea, intestinal gas, eczema, and arthritis.

Goldenseal (*Hydrastis canadensis*): Antibiotic used for colds, flu, lung disorders, coughs, all types of infections, cancer, tumors, and constipation. Blood cleanser.

Gotu Kola (*Hydrocotyle asiatica*): Stimulates the brain, improves memory, and is used for longevity and rejuvenation.

Hawthorn Berries (*Crataegus oxyacanthus*): Used for blood pressure problems, arteriosclerosis, all types of heart disorders, insomnia, nervous tension, and kidney problems.

Hops (*Humulus lupulus*): A diuretic and sedative that stimulates appetite and is used to treat insomnia, nervous conditions, pain, tension, liver trouble, and hangover.

Horsetail (*Equisetum hyemale*): A diuretic also used for broken bones, anemia, ulcers, and lung problems. Also good for skin, teeth, and hair.

Hyssop (*Hyssopus officinalis*): Useful in treating coughs, colds, bronchitis, mucous congestion, intestinal gas, asthma, lung troubles, skin eruptions, and stomach troubles. Also used as a gargle for sore throat.

Juniper Berries (*Juniperis communis*): Diuretic and antitoxin used for digestive problems, kidney and bladder disorders, and gonorrhea.

Licorice Root (*Glycyrrhiza glabra*): Diuretic and laxative, also soothes the stomach and digestive tract. Used for coughs, colds, bronchitis, congestion in lungs, and bladder and kidney ailments.

Lobelia (*Lobelia inflata*): Good for almost every ailment known, especially asthma, bronchitis, lung congestion, circulation problems, poisoning, pain, spasms, colds, lockjaw, fever, and cramps.

Mandrake (*Podophyllum peltatum*): Used for cancer, constipation, and liver troubles. Should be used with caution.

Mistletoe (*Viscum flavescens*): Strengthens the heart, increases uterine contractions; used for epilepsy, convulsions, hysteria, seizures, and nervousness.

Mugwort (*Artemisia vulgaris*): Stimulates appetite and proper digestion. Used to treat gout and rheumatism.

Mullein (*Verbascum thapsus*): Used for tuberculosis, asthma, bronchitis, cramps, earaches, pain, hay fever, and hemorrhoids.

Myrrh Gum (*Commiphora myrrha*): A skin tonic, also used for bad breath, sore gums, coughs, asthma, lung problems, ulcers, and congestion.

Nettle (*Urtica capitata*): A diuretic that stimulates digestion. Used to treat hemorrhoids and urinary disorders.

Papaya Leaf (*Carica papaya*): Supreme digestive aid that soothes the stomach, relieves allergies, digests proteins, and kills worms.

Parsley (*Petroselinum sativum*): Diuretic used for gallstones, intestinal gas, swollen glands, bad breath, kidney trouble, liver and spleen disorders, painful menstruation, anemia, and high blood pressure.

Passionflower (*Passiflora coerulea*): Used for pain relief, insomnia, headaches, nervousness, hysteria, and spasms.

Pennyroyal (*Mentha pulegium*): Useful in treating spasms, nervousness, leprosy, nausea, and headache. Stimulates menstruation. Do not use during pregnancy—may induce abortion.

Peppermint (*Mentha piperita*): Used for poor digestion, diarrhea, bowel problems, colds, flu, nausea, abdominal pains, intestinal gas, and vomiting.

Psyllium Seed (*Plantago psyllium*): Increases bowel activity; used as a cleanser by increasing intestinal bulk.

Raspberry Leaf (*Rubus idaeus*): Primarily used during pregnancy to ease delivery.

Red Clover (*Trifolium pratense*): Used for cancer, tumors, blood cleanser, syphilis, sores, leprosy, coughs, and bronchitis.

Rose Hips (*Rosa canina*): Good for colds.

Rue (*Ruta graveolens*): Useful in treating gout, rheumatic pain, intestinal gas, spasms, convulsions, hysteria, painful menstruation, eye trouble, and nervous heart afflictions.

Sage (*Salvia officinalis*): Used for sore throat, congestion, nervousness, and night sweats.

Saint-John's-Wort (*Hypericum periforatum*): Used to treat nervousness, insomnia, headache, cramps, and jaundice.

Sarsaparilla (*Similax officinalis*): Blood purifier used for all skin eruptions, colds, intestinal gas, fevers, syphilis, and impotence.

Sassafras (*Sassafras officinale*): Blood purifier, antiseptic, and diuretic, used for toothache, skin eruptions, arthritis, gout, rheumatism, and fever.

Saw Palmetto (*Serrenoa serrulata*): A general tonic used in particular for asthma, colds, bronchitis, congestion, and impotence.

Senna (*Cassia acutifolia*): Supreme cathartic useful in treating constipation.

Skullcap (*Scutellaria lateriflora*): Used for insomnia, nervousness, neuralgia, pain, hysteria, spasms, and poisonous bites.

Slippery Elm (*Ulmus fulva*): Useful in treating inflammation (internal or external), asthma, bronchitis, stomach irritation, bowel troubles, and sore throat.

Squaw Vine (*Mitchella repens*): A female regulator that facilitates childbirth. Diuretic used to treat kidney and urinary disorders.

Stoneroot (*Collinsonia canadensis*): Diuretic, used for a variety of urinary problems.

Uva Ursi (*Arctostaphylos uva-ursi*): Useful in treating kidney and bladder problems, syphilis, gonorrhea, cystitis, all urinary complaints, bronchitis, and dysentery.

Valerian (*Valeriana officinalis*): Used for pain, nervousness, insomnia, spasms, cramps, fatigue, hysteria, delirium, and neuralgia.

Virginia Snakeroot (*Aristolochia serpentaria*): A stimulant that aids digestion and is used to treat poison ivy and poisonous bites.

Wood Betony (*Betonica officinalis*): Used for headache, neuralgia, kidney and bladder problems, asthma, bronchitis, and dizziness.

Wormwood (*Artemisia absinthium*): Stimulates digestion, and is used to treat liver troubles, intestinal gas, nausea, worms, and jaundice.

Yarrow (*Archillea millefolium*): Blood purifier that induces perspiration and stimulates appetite. Used for fevers, intestinal gas, liver and gallbladder problems, and urinary disorders.

Yellow Dock (*Rumex crispus*): A blood purifier used for cancer, tumors, liver trouble, all skin problems, leprosy, syphilis, and digestive problems.

Yohimbe: An aphrodisiac.

Herbal Formula/Ailment Chart

This chart provides a list of herbal formulas, in alphabetical order according to the ailments for which they are used. Each formula is numbered for easy reference, and the full ingredients for each formula are provided. In addition, the activity of each formula is briefly described, along with recommendations for use. All of these formulas are standard herbal blends which have been developed by the leading traditional herbalists of this age. They are readily obtained at quality natural food stores, and their ingredients are listed on product labels. While there are many excellent brands of herbal formulas available, the brand with the most consistent availability and product variety is Nature's Way Herbs, of Utah. They manufacture high quality products, and supply most of the formulas described here. All capsules listed here should be taken with ample amounts of water, as directed.

Formula #1
Allergies
contains: Brigham Tea, Marshmallow Root, Burdock Root, Goldenseal Root, Chaparral, Parsley, Cayenne, and Lobelia.
activity: Used for hay fever, allergies, and sinus problems.
recommended use: Two capsules, three times daily, or as needed.

Formula #2
Antimucus Tincture
contains: Elderberry extract.
activity: Used to discharge mucus from the body, and to reduce cysts.
recommended use: Three drops in a cup of warm water, or as needed.

Formula #3
Antiseptic Ointment
contains: Comfrey Leaves, Marshmallow Root, Marigold, Blue Malva Flowers, Chickweed, Mullein, Plantain, Natural Oils, Beeswax.
activity: For burns, bruises, lesions, abrasions, scaling, inflammation, and poison ivy.
recommended use: Apply externally as desired.

Formula #4
Antispasmodic and Nerve Tincture
contains: Extracts of Skullcap, Lobelia, Valerian Root, Myrrh Gum, Black Cohosh, Cayenne.
activity: For tremors, cramps, fainting, hysteria, delirium, nervousness.
recommended use: Three drops in a cup of hot herb tea, three times daily.

154/HERBOLOGY

Formula #5
Arthritis, Rheumatism
contains: Yucca concentrate, Hydrangea, Brigham Tea, Burdock Root, Chaparral, Black Walnut Leaves, Wild Lettuce, Sarsaparilla Root, Wormwood, Valerian Root, Lobelia, Cayenne, Black Cohosh, Chelated Minerals.
activity: To reduce swelling and inflammation in joints and connective tissue, and to relieve pain and stiffness.
recommended use: Start with one capsule twice daily, and gradually increase to two capsules three times daily.

Formula #6
Asthma Syrup
contains: Comfrey Root, Mullein, Garlic, Fennel Seed, Lobelia, Vegetable Glycerine, Apple Cider Vinegar.
activity: To expell mucus from throat, bronchial tubes, and lungs, and to relieve muscle spasms and asthmatic coughing.
recommended use: One teaspoonful, three times daily.

Formula #7
Blood Cleanser
contains: Gentian, Allheal, Catnip, Goldenseal Root, Bayberry Bark, Myrrh Gum, Irish Moss, Fenugreek, Comfrey Root, Bugleweed, Yellow Dock Root, Saint-Johns-Wort, Blue Vervain, Prickly Ash Berries, Violet Leaves, Stillingia, Red Clover Blossoms, Cascara Sagrada Bark, Chickweed, Cyani Flowers.
activity: Removes toxic waste from the body, thereby cleaning the bloodstream. Powerful total systemic cleanser.
recommended use: Two capsules, three times daily, or as needed.

Formula #8
Blood Pressure (low or high)
contains: Cayenne, Parsley, Ginger Root, Goldenseal Root, Garlic, Siberian Ginseng.
activity: To normalize either high or low blood pressure, and to enhance circulation.
recommended use: Two or more capsules twice daily.

Formula #9
Blood Pressure (high)
contains: Cayenne, Garlic.
activity: To lower high blood pressure to normal level. Also improves circulation and digestion.
recommended use: Two capsules, three times daily.

Formula #10
Blood Purification, Detoxification

contains: Red Clover Blossoms, Chaparral, Licorice Root, Peach Bark, Oregon Grape Root, Stillingia, Cascara Sagrada Bark, Sarsaparilla Root, Prickly Ash Bark, Burdock Root, Buckthorn Bark.
activity: A total systemic cleanser, also used in the treatment of cancer.
recommended use: Two capsules, three times daily.

Formula #11
Bone, Flesh, Cartilage Builder
contains: White Oak Bark, Comfrey Root, Marshmallow Root, Mullein, Black Walnut Hulls, Gravel Root, Wormwood, Lobelia, Skullcap.
activity: To heal broken bones, sprains, and damaged cartilage.
recommended use: Two capsules, three times daily.

Formula #12
Bowel Function
contains: Wheat Bran, Papaya Leaves.
activity: Enhances digestion and promotes regularity.
recommended use: Two capsules with every meal.

Formula #13
Colds, Coughs
contains: Fenugreek Seed, Comfrey Leaves.
activity: Breaks up congestive mucus, and helps to restore breathing.
recommended use: Two capsules each morning and evening.

Formula #14
Colds, Flu
contains: Garlic, Rose Hips, Parsley, Watercress, Rosemary.
activity: Helps relieve the symptoms of colds and flu.
recommended use: Two or more capsules, morning and evening.

Formula #15
Cold and Flu Syrup
contains: Comfrey Root, Wormwood, Lobelia, Marshmallow Root, White Oak Bark, Black Walnut Bark, Mullein, Skullcap, Uva-Ursi, Apple Cider Vinegar, Vegetable Glycerine, Honey, Garlic Juice.
activity: Natural antibiotic, useful in preventing or treating colds, flu.
recommended use: One teaspoon, three times daily.

Formula #16
Cold Prevention
contains: Bayberry Bark, Ginger Root, Cloves, Cayenne, White Pine Bark.
activity: To prevent colds, and to relieve cold symptoms quickly.
recommended use: Two capsules, three times daily or as needed.

156/Herbology

Formula #17
Cough Syrup
contains: Chickweed, Licorice Root, Comfrey Root, Mullein, Marshmallow Root, Horehound, Lobelia, Cayenne, Vegetable Glycerine.
activity: To relieve coughs, congestion, and hoarseness.
recommended use: One teaspoonful, as needed.

Formula #18
Digestive Aid
contains: Comfrey Leaf, Pepsin
activity: To assist protein digestion, and to break down accumulated mucus in the digestive tract.
recommended use: Two capsules, three times daily.

Formula #19
Digestive Disorders
contains: Comfrey Leaves, Cayenne, Papain.
activity: A general aid to digestion.
recommended use: Two or more capsules, morning and evening.

Formula #20
Ear Tincture
contains: Extracts of Black Cohosh, Blue Cohosh, Blue Vervain, Scullcap, Lobelia.
activity: Used to relieve ear infections and to restore equilibrium.
recommended use: Three or more drops orally, or apply as needed.

Formula #21
Energy, Endurance, Stamina
contains: Ginseng
activity: Enhances the body's energy production mechanisms.
recommended use: Two or more capsules daily.

Formula #22
Eye Disorders
contains: Eyebright, Goldenseal Root, Bayberry Bark, Red Raspberry Leaves, Cayenne.
activity: For strengthening the eyes, healing lesions, and dissolving cataracts.
recommended use: Two or more capsules, twice daily.

Formula #23
Fatigue, Stress, Debility
contains: Siberian Ginseng, Gotu Kola, Cayenne.
activity: For energy, stamina, alertness, immunity, detoxification, and overall fortification.

recommended use: Two capsules, three times daily.

Formula #24
Fever, Flu
contains: Fenugreek Seed, Thyme.
activity: To reduce fever and eliminate congestion.
recommended use: Two capsules, morning and evening.

Formula #25
Gland Problems
contains: Mullein, Lobelia.
activity: Effective for glandular malfunction, and to reduce swollen lymphatic glands.
recommended use: Two capsules, twice daily.

Formula #26
Glands (swollen, infected lymph)
contains: Plantain, Black Walnut Leaves, Goldenseal Root, Marshmallow Root, Bugleweed, Lobelia.
activity: To cleanse swollen lymph nodes and fight infection.
recommended use: Two capsules, twice daily.

Formula #27
Glandular Infections
contains: Echinacea, Goldenseal Root, Cayenne.
activity: Antibacterial, antibiotic, useful for lymphatic, glandular, and ear infections.
recommended use: Two capsules, twice daily.

Formula #28
Heart
contains: Hawthorn Berries, Cayenne, Vitamin E, Lecithin.
activity: To reduce serum cholesterol, enhance circulation, and promote total cardiovascular function.
recommended use: One capsule in the morning and evening.

Formula #29
Hormonal Imbalances
contains: Black Cohosh, Sarsaparilla Root, Siberian Ginseng, Licorice Root, False Unicorn, Blessed Thistle, Squaw Vine.
activity: For proper pituitary, pancreatic, and glandular function, for hormonal balance. Valuable during puberty, pregnancy, and menopause. Useful for both men and women.
recommended use: Two capsules, morning and evening.

Formula #30
Hypoglycemia
contains: Licorice Root, Cedar Berries, Juniper Berries, Wild Yam, Dandelion Root, Pumpkin Seed.
activity: To aid in restoring normal blood sugar level in case of hypoglycemia. Acts upon pancreas, adrenals, and liver.
recommended use: Two capsules, three times daily.

Formula #31
Impotence
contains: Damiana, Siberian Ginseng, Echinacea, Fo-Ti, Gotu Kola, Sarsaparilla Root, Saw Palmetto.
activity: Enhances libido and sexual function.
recommended use: Two capsules, three times daily.

Formula #32
Insomnia
contains: Hops Flowers, Valerian Root, Skullcap.
activity: Promotes sleep.
recommended use: Two or more capsules prior to retiring.

Formula #33
Kidney and Bladder
contains: Juniper Berries, Parsley, Uva Ursi, Marshmallow Root, Lobelia, Ginger Root, Goldenseal Root.
activity: Heals and strengthens kidneys and bladder, eliminates toxins and waste from kidneys, bladder, and urethra.
recommended use: Two capsules, morning and evening.

Formula #34
Kidney Function
contains: Garlic and Parsley.
activity: Enhances urination, detoxifies kidneys.
recommended use: Two capsules, morning and evening.

Formula #35
Laxative
contains: Senna Leaves, Buckthorn Bark, Licorice Root, Alfalfa Leaves, Fennel Seed, Aniseed, Malva Flowers, Culver's Root, Turkey Rhubarb Root.
activity: Relieves occasional constipation.
recommended use: Two or more tablets before bed.

Formula #36
Liver, Gallbladder

contains: Barberry Root Bark, Wild Yam, Crampbark, Fennel Seed, Ginger Root, Catnip, Peppermint.
activity: To enhance liver and gallbladder function, for detoxification, and to stimulate the flow of bile.
recommended use: Two capsules, three times daily, prior to meals.

Formula #37
Lower Bowel Tonic and Cleanser
contains: Cascara Sagrada Bark, Barberry Root Bark, Cayenne, Ginger Root, Goldenseal Root, Lobelia, Red Raspberry Leaves, Turkey Rhubarb Root, Fennel Seed.
activity: Activates the lower bowel, eliminates old, accumulated waste, helps to rebuild the bowel, and enhances normal function.
recommended use: Two capsules, three times daily.

Formula #38
Memory Aid
contains: Blue Vervain, Blessed Thistle, Gotu Kola, Lobelia, Cayenne, Ginger Root.
activity: To enhance memory and mental alertness.
recommended use: Two capsules, three times daily.

Formula #39
Menstrual Regulator
contains: Goldenseal Root, Blessed Thistle, Cayenne, Uva Ursi Leaves, Crampbark, False Unicorn, Red Raspberry Leaves, Squaw Vine, Ginger Root.
activity: To regulate menstruation, and to relieve swelling and cramping.
recommended use: Two capsules, three times daily.

Formula #40
Nervous Disorders
contains: Black Cohosh, Cayenne, Hops Flowers, Mistletoe, Lobelia, Skullcap, Wood Betony, Valerian Root, Lady's Slipper.
activity: Relaxes, soothes, and calms the nerves. Also good for insomnia.
recommended use: Two capsules, two or three times daily.

Formula #41
Pain, Headaches
contains: Wild Lettuce, Valerian Root, Cayenne.
activity: For pain relief, and as an aid for nervous tension and headaches.
recommended use: Two capsules, three times daily.

Formula #42
Pain Tincture

contains: Extracts of Wild Lettuce, Valerian Root.
activity: Soothes and calms nerves, relieves pain.
recommended use: Three drops in a cup of hot herb tea.

Formula #43
Pancreas
contains: Cedar Berries, Uva Ursi Leaves, Licorice Root, Mullein, Cayenne, Goldenseal Root.
activity: An aid to maintaining and restoring proper pancreatic function.
recommended use: Two capsules, three times daily.

Formula #44
Parasites
contains: Pumpkin Seed, Culver's Root, Violet Leaves, Cascara Sagrada Bark, Comfrey Root, Slippery Elm Bark, Witch Hazel Bark, Mullein, Echinacea.
activity: Destroys and eliminates internal parasites.
recommended use: Three or more capsules, three times daily.

Formula #45
Pre-natal Formula
contains: Squaw Vine, Blessed Thistle, Black Cohosh, Pennyroyal, False Unicorn, Red Raspberry Leaves, Lobelia.
activity: Prepares a mother's body for easier delivery.
recommended use: Six weeks prior to delivery, start with two capsules, four times daily. For last two weeks, take three capsules, four times daily.

Formula #46
Prostate, Kidney
contains: Cayenne, Uva Ursi Leaves, Parsley, Goldenseal Root, Gravel Root, Juniper Berries, Marshmallow Root, Ginger Root, Korean White Ginseng.
activity: To relieve inflammation or infection of the prostate, and to break down kidney stones.
recommended use: Two capsules, three times daily.

Formula #47
Respiratory Aid
contains: Marshmallow Root, Mullein, Comfrey Leaves, Lobelia, Chickweed.
activity: Clears and heals the entire respiratory tract.
recommended use: Two or more capsules, three times daily.

Formula #48
Skin Aid
contains: Alfalfa Leaves, Kelp, Dandelion Root.

activity: Useful for treatment of acne, itching, scaling, and inflammation of the skin.
recommended use: Two capsules, three times daily.

Formula #49
Skin Blemishes
contains: Dandelion Root, Sassafras, Burdock Root, Licorice Root, Echinacea, Yellow Dock Root, Kelp, Cayenne, Chaparral.
activity: For thorough cleansing of the body, to eliminate pimples, cysts, and other skin eruptions indicative of accumulated internal waste and debris.
recommended use: Two capsules, three times daily.

Formula #50
Spring Tonic
contains: Sassafras, Gotu Kola, Catnip, Dandelion Root, Chickweed, Yellow Dock Root, Siberian Ginseng.
activity: A general cleanser to revitalize the body in springtime.
recommended use: Two capsules, morning and evening.

Formula #51
Stomach Tincture
contains: Extracts of Catnip and Fennel Seed.
activity: Relieves minor stomach spasms, pains, and gas, and soothes indigestion. Good for colic also.
recommended use: Three to six drops in a cup of water.

Formula #52
Teeth and Gums
contains: Horsetail Grass, White Oak Bark, Oat Straw, Comfrey Root, Peppermint, Cloves, Lobelia.
activity: Cleans and whitens teeth, strengthens gums.
recommended use: As a tooth powder. Use to brush daily.

Formula #53
Thyroid
contains: Mullein, Parsley, Watercress, Kelp, Irish Moss, Iceland Moss, Lobelia.
activity: Feeds and nourishes the thyroid, thereby assisting in the balance of metabolism.
recommended use: Two capsules, three times daily.

Formula #54
Ulcers
contains: Myrrh Gum, Goldenseal Root, Cayenne.

162/Herbology

activity: Active materials heal ulcers, infections, burns, cuts, wounds, bruises, sprains.
recommended use: Two capsules, three times daily.

Formula #55
Weight Control
contains: Chickweed, Saffron, Burdock Root, Parsley, Kelp, Licorice Root, Fennel Seed, Echinacea, Black Walnut Leaves, Papaya Leaves, Hawthorn Berries.
activity: Assists in bowel cleansing, diminishing appetite, and burning fat.
recommended use: Two capsules, 30 minutes prior to each meal.

Herbal Tea Bag/Ailment Chart

This chart is a short list of herbal tea formulas already available in tea bag form. These products are made by Traditional Medicinals of Rohnert Park, California, and are actually over-the-counter drugs, even though they contain only all natural herbs. These teas are readily obtained at quality natural food stores. Their names and ingredients are the same as the ones given here. Each formula is effective, and very easy to prepare.

Formula #56
Breathe Easy Herbal Decongestant
contains: Ma Huang, Peppermint Leaf, Licorice Root, Marigold Flowers, Fennel Seeds, Ginger Root, Eucalyptus Leaf, Pleurisy Root, Coltsfoot Leaf.
activity: Relieves bronchial and nasal congestion, stuffy nose and wheezing associated with bronchial asthma, the common cold, hay fever, sinusitis, and other respiratory allergies.
recommended use: At the first sign of discomfort, drink one to two cups every four hours, not to exceed eight cups in 24 hours.

Formula #57
Gypsy Cold Care Herb Cold Medicine
contains: Peppermint Leaf, Cinnamon Bark, Orange peel, Coltsfoot Leaf, Safflower, Hyssop, Ginger Root, Clove Stems, Rose Hips, Elder Flowers, Stevia Leaf.
activity: Relieves nasal congestion and stuffy nose and helps relieve coughs due to minor throat and bronchial irritation associated with the common cold.
recommended use: One to two cups at the first sign of cold discomfort and then every three hours, not to exceed eight cups in 24 hours.

Formula #58
Smoker's Tea Smoking Deterrent
contains: Lobelia, Peppermint Leaf, Clove Stems, Eucalyptus Leaf, Orange Peel,

Althea Root, Licorice Root, Red Clover Blossom, Stevia Leaf, Ascorbic Acid (vitamin C).
activity: An aid to stop smoking. Helps curb the craving for nicotine.
recommended use: Drink one cup every hour, not to exceed 12 cups in 24 hours.

Formula #59
Smooth Move Herbal Laxative
contains: Cascara Sagrada, Senna Leaf, Orange Peel, Licorice Root, Ginger Root, Fennel Seeds, Cinnamon Bark, Flaxseeds.
activity: For relieving occasional constipation.
recommended use: Drink one half to one cup before bed time.

Formula #60
Throat Coat Soothes Sore Throats
contains: Slippery Elm Bark, Wild Cherry Bark, Licorice Root, Fennel Seeds, Cinnamon Bark, Orange Peel, Althea Root.
activity: Provides temporary relief from minor discomfort of sore, irritated and raw throats due to colds, smoking, prolonged speaking, or exposure to dampness.
recommended use: Drink at the first signs of throat discomfort. Repeat every two hours as needed.

Formula #61
Weightless Tea Herbal Diet Aid
contains: Uva Ursi Leaf, Fennel Seeds, Lemon Verbena, Hibiscus Flowers, Lemon Grass Leaf, Flaxseeds, Red Clover Blossoms, Cleavers Herb, Stevia Leaf, Buchu Leaf.
activity: Helps curb appetite, and assists in relieving temporary water weight gain.
recommended use: One to two cups between meals, not to exceed eight cups in 24 hours.

Special Herbal Extracts and Tablets

Though the purpose of this book is not to be a showcase of commercial herbal products per se, I have the unique opportunity to recommend those few available items which are excellent above and beyond all common standards. Among such an elite group are the rare and exotic products made by Yellow Emperor, and East Earth Herbs. For the person who is serious about generating health and vitality, or for the health practitioner who is ever on the lookout for the most valuable products, these items will satisfy all criteria. They are included here for your benefit, to further your adventures on the road to ever-increasing inner balance, personal power, and fulfillment.

164/ HERBOLOGY

YELLOW EMPEROR FORMULAS: These liquid extracts are available in natural food stores. They are quite powerful, and produce significant results.

Formula #62
Shiu Chu Ginseng Extract: This is recommended for use when the body is depleted, such as after a long illness. It is also useful when an excessive amount of energy is required. This intensely strong ginseng extract should be used only occasionally.

Formula #63
East-West Blend: Oriental Ginseng and American Woods-grown ginseng together create a balanced ginseng formula which offers stimulation and endurance, without a sudden "let-down." Excellent for athletes and active people, for regular use.

Formula #64
Siberian Ginseng: This extract helps increase mental clarity and physical stamina, particularly under stressful conditions, while also building resistance to disease. Siberian Ginseng is valuable for increasing one's capacity to work, and for fighting stress.

Formula #65
Wild American Ginseng: Prized by Americans and Orientals alike, this is one of the world's rarest ginsengs. Wild American Ginseng is highly potent, stimulating the brain, energy production, and immunity. Because of its rarity, it is costly—and worth it.

Formula #66
Woodsgrown Ginseng: Another high quality Ginseng, this American variety is not wild, but grown free of chemicals nonetheless, in the woods. It is highly potent, yet more available than the Wild variety. Its properties are similar.

Formula #67
Dong Quai: This Oriental herb is traditionally known for its use as a female regulator, to relieve menstrual cramping, and to alleviate many of the discomforts associated with menopause. In extract form it is absorbed and utilized quickly and effectively.

Formula #68
Fo-Ti: This gentle herb has been used by the Chinese for centuries, as a tonic for the kidneys, liver, blood, pancreas, spleen, and brain. It is complementary to ginseng, and enhances the activity of that herb. It is an overall health-builder, and can be used daily.

Formula #69
Ginger: This extract is an excellent remedy for motion sickness, and is useful in alleviating discomfort due to stomach flu, overeating, and indigestion.

Formula #70
Goldenseal: This versatile herb has anticongestive, antibiotic properties. It is useful in cases of colds and flu, internal and external inflammations, intestinal disorders, sore gums, cuts and wounds.

EAST EARTH HERBS: These formulas are based on the Oriental understanding of energy balancing. They are available in both tablet and extract form, at quality natural food stores.

Formula #71
Dragon Brew: This beverage is useful for sustained energy, health of internal organs, general vitality, improved circulation, strong digestion, regularity, mental clarity, and total balance. It can be used daily.

Formula #72
Shiu Chu Ginseng: Because this is the most powerful, energy-producing ginseng available, it is for those who are depleted, or for those times when a very high energy state is required. This is not a product to be taken daily, but to be used occasionally, as needed.

Formula #73
Tang Kuei: Also known as Dong Quai, this herb is traditionally known as a female regulator, to relieve menstrual cramping, and to alleviate many of the discomforts associated with menopause.

Formula #74
Express: Providing a fast acting energy lift as well as a sustained energy level, Express is an excellent substitute for caffeine beverages, as it not only gets you going, but nourishes the body as well. Express increases one's capacity for work and productivity.

Formula #75
Women's Longevity: This woman's formula balances a woman's cycle, and nourishes the kidneys, liver, spleen, and heart. It is, above all, a supremely nourishing formula, balancing the subtle and delicate forces within a woman.

Formula #76
Four Ginsengs: This ginseng blend provides a smooth, balanced energy that is steady and even. It does not produce a dramatic lift, but rather gently guides the body to a higher level of performance, gradually. The formula nourishes the liver, heart, stomach, lungs, and kidneys.

Formula #77
Peaceful: While not a sedative, Peaceful enables one to achieve a deep, satisfying feeling of inner peace and calm, without deadening the senses. Peaceful enables one to let go of excessive energies, and achieve a state of ease.

Formula #78
Sage's Ginseng: This rare wild mountain Ginseng from the interior of China is unlike any other herbal product available. It dramatically enhances brain function and mental clarity, and is fabulous for meditation. The refined energy achieved with use of this ginseng formula lifts the body/mind to a highly sophisticated and subtle strata.

YOGATHERAPY REPERTORY

How to Use the Yogatherapy Repertory

In the previous five chapters of this book, there is detailed information about Yoga (Chapter 1), Ingredients of Natural Living (Chapter 2), Nutrition (Chapter 3), Vitamins, Minerals, and Food Supplements (Chapter 4), and Herbology (Chapter 5). Each of these chapters may be used separately. If you are just interested in the therapeutic effects of Yoga postures, you can study Chapter 1 by itself, without ever involving yourself with the herbal pharmacology of Chapter 5. However, if you wish to tie all of the material in the first five chapters together, then the Yogatherapy Repertory will be of great value to you.

The Yogatherapy Repertory is a list of 54 health conditions and a comprehensive, recommended plan for each one. For each condition, there are recommendations for Yoga Postures, Foods, a Juice Formula, Supplements, Herb Teas, and Herbal Formulas. Not every condition is a disorder. Two cases in point are Pregnancy and Rejuvenation. Most of the conditions listed, however, are actual health problems. You will notice that many of the conditions are extremely broad. "Bladder Disorders" or "Thyroid Disorders" are general headings. For both the bladder and the thyroid there are actually hundreds of specific ailments. However, the Yogatherapy Repertory is not intended to be used as specific therapy for specific diseases. Rather, it is designed for use as a holistic support program for broad categories of needs.

To use the Yogatherapy Repertory, look up the condition which most interests you. Under the heading **Yoga Postures**, you will find a list of postures, given in the order that they are presented in Chapter 1. Refer back to Chapter 1, and you will learn exactly how to perform each technique.

Under the heading **Foods**, recommendations are given for dietary modifications. To find out more about the recommendations listed, refer back to Chapter 3, Nutrition. There you will find specific information about the Yogatherapy Cleansing Program, the Yogatherapy Diet, Lemon Water Fasting, and specific categories of foods.

Under the heading **Juice Formula,** you will find a specific formula for a vegetable or fruit juice combination. More information about juices and how to prepare them can be found in Chapter 3, Nutrition.

Under the heading **Supplements**, you will find a list of vitamins, minerals, and food supplements, and recommended dosages. While this list is complete in and of itself, you may wish to know more about the supplements listed. If so, you will find that information in Chapter 4, Vitamins, Minerals, and Food Supplements.

Under the heading **Herb Teas**, you will find a list of individual herb teas recommended for the particular health condition on that page. More detailed information on each herb listed, along with an explanation of how to prepare herb teas, can be found in Chapter 5, Herbology.

Under the heading **Herbal Formulas**, you will find a list of numbers. Each is the number of a specific herbal formula which is fully described in Chapter 5, Herbology. In Chapter 5, the herbal formulas are listed by number, for quick reference.

The supplements, herbs, and herbal formulas listed and described here are all available in quality natural food stores. I have made every effort to list those products and categories of products which are most readily available.

The Yogatherapy Repertory is a convenient, easy to use reference which can be of great value in the creation of a personalized health program. May it serve you well.

Acne

Yoga Postures:

Soorya Namaskar, Rejuvenation Series, Triangle Pose, Standing Leg Stretch, Palm to Floor Pose, Forward Knee Pose, Supine Spinal Twist, Pelvic Pose, *Mahamudra* 1, 2, 3, Peacock Pose, Reverse Seal.

Foods:

Yogatherapy Cleansing Program, Yogatherapy Diet, especially papaya, fresh green vegetables, brewer's yeast. Reduce intake of fats, oils, and dairy products until condition has improved.

Juice Formula:

carrot 6 oz., spinach 4 oz., parsley 2 oz.

Supplements:

Beta-Carotene 25,000 I.U.
B-complex 50 mg.
B_1 100 mg.
B_2 100 mg.
C with Bioflavonoids 2–4 grams
High Potency Multi Minerals
Niacin 50 mg.
E 400 I.U.
Kelp 3 tablets
Zinc 25–50 mg.

Herb Teas:

Burdock Root, Chaparral, Comfrey Leaf, Elecampane, Golden Seal, Horsetail, Hyssop, Parsley, Red Clover, Sarsaparilla, Sassafras, Yellow Dock.

Herbal Formulas:

#7, #10, #48, #49

Adenoids, Tonsils

Yoga Postures:

Neck Pose, Standing Back Stretch, Forward Knee Pose, Forward Knee Pose w/ Back Stretch, Forward Knee/Palm Pose, Fish Pose, Cobra Pose, Bridge Pose, Shoulder Stand.

Foods:

During inflammation, lemon water fast. Yogatherapy Diet, especially fresh raw vegetables and fruits. Be conservative with intake of dairy products.

Juice Formula:

carrot 10 oz., parsley 2 oz., 2 cloves garlic (omit garlic if formula is given to children)

Supplements:

C with Bioflavonoids 2–6 grams
A 10,000–25,000 I.U.
Beta-Carotene 25,000 I.U.
Pantothenic Acid 250 mg.
B-complex 50 mg.
Kyolic Liquid 1/2 tsp. 3 times daily
Kelp 3 tablets

Herb Teas:

Bayberry, Burdock Root, Chickweed, Coltsfoot, Comfrey Leaf or Root, Echinacea, Elecampane, Eucalyptus, Fenugreek, Ginger, Goldenseal, Hyssop, Lobelia, Mullein, Slippery Elm. Also, cayenne, garlic in food.

Herbal Formulas:

#14–16, #57, #60

Alcoholism, Drug Addiction

Yoga Postures:

Soorya Namaskar, Rejuvenation Series, Triangle Pose, Knee to Chest Pose, Moving Knee to Chest Pose, Supine Spinal Twist, Pelvic Pose, Lotus Pose, *Mahamudra* 1, 2, 3, Inclined Spinal Twist, Bow Pose, Cobra Pose, Peacock Pose, Reverse Seal.

Foods:

40-Day-Yogatherapy-Cleansing-Program, Yogatherapy Diet, especially beets, carrots, leafy greens, salads, whole grains, plenty of juices, brewer's yeast. Repeated lemon water fasts.

Juice Formula:

carrot 8 oz., beet 4 oz.,
OR
carrot 4 oz., celery 4 oz., parsley 2 oz., spinach 2 oz.

Supplements:

A 25,000 I.U.
B-complex 100 mg.
Niacin 100 mg.
N, N, Dimethylglycine (DMG) 100 mg.
Brewer's Yeast 2 Tbsp.
C with Bioflavonoids 2–6 grams
Multiple Digestive Enzymes 1 tablet with each meal for 2 months
E 400–800 I.U.
L-Glutamine 2–5 grams

Herb Teas:

Agrimony, Barberry, Bayberry, Burdock Root, Chaparral, Comfrey Leaf or Root, Dandelion, Ginseng, Goldenseal, Gotu Kola, Lobelia, Parsley, Red Clover, Sarsaparilla, Sassafras, Yarrow, Yellow Dock.

Herbal Formulas:

#7, #10, #36, #62, #71

Allergies, Hay Fever

Yoga Postures:

Palm Pose, Neck Pose, Standing Back Stretch, Forward Knee Pose, Forward Knee Pose with Back Stretch, Forward Knee/Palm Pose, Lion Pose, Lotus Spinal Stretch, Camel Pose, Wheel Pose.

Foods:

Short lemon water fasts, Yogatherapy Cleansing Program during allergy periods. Yogatherapy Diet, especially fresh juices. Eliminate milk products and reduce intake of eggs until condition has cleared.

Juice Formula:

carrot 8 oz., cucumber 2 oz., beet 2 oz.,
OR
celery 4 oz., spinach 4 oz., parsley 2 oz., radish 2 oz.

Supplements:

A 10,000–25,000 I.U.
C with Bioflavonoids 2–6 grams
D 400–1,000 I.U.
E 400 I.U.
High Potency Multi Minerals
Kelp 3–10 tablets
Multiple Digestive Enzymes 1 with each meal for 2 months
Pantothenic Acid 1–2 grams

Herb Teas:

Coltsfoot, Comfrey Leaf or Root, Elecampane, Eucalyptus, Goldenseal, Hyssop, Licorice Root, Lobelia, Mullein, Myrrh Gum, Sage. Also, cayenne and garlic in food.

Herbal Formulas:

#1, #2, #10, #56, #70

Anemia

Yoga Postures:

Soorya Namaskar, Rejuvenation Series, Palm to Floor Pose, Inverted Leg Pose, Pelvic Pose, Rock Pose, Lotus Pose, Lotus Spinal Stretch, *Mahamudra* 1, 2, 3, Inclined Pose, Wheel Pose.

Foods:

Yogatherapy Diet, especially nuts, seeds, seafood, whole grains, leafy green vegetables, sprouts, brewer's yeast, foods high in B_{12} and iron.

Juice Formula:

carrot 6 oz., beet 3 oz., spinach 3 oz.

Supplements:

A 10,000–25,000 I.U.
B-complex 50 mg.
B_{12} 500 mcg.
Brewer's Yeast 2 Tbsp.
C with Bioflavonoids 2–4 grams
Folic Acid 400 mcg.
Calcium 1,000 mg.
Iron 30 mg.
High Potency Multi Minerals

Herb Teas:

Alfalfa, Burdock Root, Chia Seed, Ginger, Ginseng, Gotu Kola, Horsetail, Parsley.

Herbal Formulas:

#62–66, #69, #71, #76

Appetite (poor, lack of)

Yoga Postures:

Soorya Namaskar, Rejuvenation Series, Knee to Chest Pose, Rock Pose, *Mahamudra* 1, 2, 3, Locust Pose, Boat Pose, Bow Pose, Camel Pose.

Foods:

Yogatherapy Diet, especially leafy greens, fresh juices, papaya, pineapple.

Juice Formula:

pineapple 12 oz.,
OR
pineapple 8 oz., ginger 1 oz.,
OR
celery 6 oz., spinach 4 oz., parsley 2 oz.

Supplements:

B-complex 50 mg.
C with Bioflavonoids 2 grams
Kelp 3–6 tablets
Alfalfa 5 tablets
MegaDophilus 1/4 tsp., 2 times daily
Bee Pollen 1/2 tsp.
High Potency Multi Minerals
Zinc 25 mg.

Herb Teas:

Alfalfa, Barberry, Bayberry, Comfrey Leaf or Root, Elecampane, Ginger, Mugwort, Nettle, Papaya Leaf, Peppermint, Slippery Elm, Yarrow.

Herbal Formulas:

#18, #19, #69, #71

Arterial Disease

Yoga Postures:

Palm Pose, One Legged Pose, Triangle Pose, Side Stretch, Forward Knee Pose, Forward Knee/Palm Pose, Pointing Pose, Rock Pose, Inclined Spinal Twist.

Foods:

Yogatherapy Cleansing Program. Yogatherapy Cleansing Diet, especially onions, garlic, leafy greens, sprouts, okra, pineapple, nonfat milk products.

Juice Formula:

celery 4 oz., spinach 4 oz., lettuce 2 oz., parsley 2 oz.

Supplements:

Niacin 100–250 mg.
C with Bioflavonoids 2–6 grams
E 400–800 I.U.
Lecithin Granules 2 Tbsp.
MaxEPA 5 capsules
Kelp 3 tablets
Brewer's Yeast 2 Tbsp.
Alfalfa 4 tablets or more tablets

Herb Teas:

Alfalfa, Burdock Root, Hawthorn Berries, Lobelia, Parsley. Also cayenne and garlic in food.

Herbal Formulas:

#7–10

Arthritis, Gout, Rheumatism

Yoga Postures:
Soorya Namaskar, Rejuvenation Series, and any other postures that you can practice comfortably.

Foods:

Yogatherapy Cleansing Program. Yogatherapy Diet, especially green salads, fresh fruits, sprouts, whole grains, olive oil.

Juice Formula:

carrot 8 oz., spinach 4 oz.,
OR
grapefruit 6 oz., celery 6 oz.,
OR
celery 4 oz., spinach 4 oz., lettuce 2 oz., parsley 2 oz.

Supplements:

C with Bioflavonoids 2–6 grams
E 400 I.U.
B-complex 50 mg.
Niacin 50 mg.
Brewer's Yeast 2 Tbsp.
Kelp 3–6 tablets
Alfalfa 6 tablets, 3 times daily
High Potency Multi Minerals

Herb Teas:

Alfalfa, Black Cohosh, Chaparral, Comfrey Leaf or Root, Devil's Claw, Goldenrod, Mugwort, Rue, Sassafras.

Herbal Formulas:

#5

Back Pain

Yoga Postures:

The Squat, Wide Squat, Palm Pose, One Legged Pose, Triangle Pose, Side Stretch, Standing Leg Stretch, Knee to Chest Pose, Supine Knee to Chest Pose, Wind Eliminating Pose, Inverted Leg Pose, Supine Spinal Twist, Easy Pose, Rock Pose, Hero Pose, Lotus Pose, Butterfly Pose, Grasshopper Pose, Plow Pose.

Foods:

Yogatherapy Diet

Juice Formula:

celery 6 oz., beet 3 oz., parsley 2 oz., ginger 1 oz.

Supplements:

B-complex 50 mg.
Brewer's Yeast 2 Tbsp.
Calcium 1,000 mg.
Zinc 25–50 mg.
Kelp 3–6 tablets
High Potency Multi Vitamin
High Potency Multi Mineral
C with Bioflavonoids 2–4 grams

Herb Teas:

Black Cohosh, Catnip, Chamomile, Comfrey Leaf or Root, Devil's Claw, Horsetail, Lobelia, Mullein, Passionflower, Pennyroyal, Rue, Skullcap, Valerian.

Herbal Formulas:

#41, #42

Bladder Disorders

Yoga Postures:

The Squat, Wide Squat, Forward Knee Pose, Seminal Control Pose, Supine Knee to Chest Pose, Celibate Pose, Crotch Stretch, Pelvic Pose, Hero Pose, Grasshopper Pose, Bow Pose, Cobra Pose.

Foods:

Yogatherapy Cleansing Program. Yogatherapy Diet, especially watermelon, pineapple, berries, coconut, leafy greens, garlic, onions, fresh green juices.

Juice Formula:

carrot 4 oz., celery 4 oz., spinach 4 oz.

Supplements:

A 10,000–25,000 I.U.
C with Bioflavonoids 2–6 grams
D 400–1,000 I.U.
High Potency Multi Mineral
Kelp 3–6 tablets

Herb Teas:

Alfalfa, Burdock Root, Chaparral, Goldenrod, Juniper Berries, Nettle, Parsley, Squaw Vine, Stoneroot, Uva Ursi, Wood Betony, Yarrow.

Herbal Formulas:

#33

Blood Pressure, High

Yoga Postures:

The Squat, Palm Pose, Forward Knee Pose, Pointing Pose, Easy Pose, Rock Pose, Hero Pose, Lotus Pose, Lotus Spinal Stretch, Corpse Pose.

Foods:

Yogatherapy Diet, especially leafy greens, fresh juices. Use nonfat dairy products.

Juice Formula:

carrot 6 oz., spinach 4 oz., parsley 2 oz., garlic 2 cloves.

Supplements:

A 10,000–25,000 I.U.
B-complex 50 mg.
E 400–800 I.U.
High Potency Multi Mineral
Calcium 1,000 mg.
Lecithin Granules 2 Tbsp.
Niacin 50–250 mg.
Kelp 3–6 tablets
MaxEPA 3–5 capsules

Herb Teas:

Alfalfa, Blue Cohosh, Parsley. Also cayenne and garlic in food.

Herbal Formulas:

#8, #9

Blood Pressure, Low

Yoga Postures:

Soorya Namaskar, Rejuvenation Series, Plow Pose, Reverse Seal, Shoulder Stand.

Foods:

Yogatherapy Diet, especially brewer's yeast, leafy greens, seafood.

Juice Formula:

carrot 8 oz., cucumber 2 oz., beet 2 oz.

Supplements:

A 10,000–25,000 i.u.
B-complex 50 mg.
E 400 i.u.
High Potency Multi Mineral
Calcium 1,000 mg.
Lecithin Granules 2 Tbsp.
Niacin 50–250 mg.
Kelp 3–6 tablets
N,N,Dimethylglycine (DMG) 100 mg.
Bee Pollen 1/2 tsp.

Herb Teas:

Alfalfa, Ginger, Ginseng, Horsetail.

Herbal Formulas:

♯8

Bronchitis

Yoga Postures:

Palm Pose, Neck Pose, Standing Back Stretch, Forward Knee Pose, Forward Knee Pose with Back Stretch, Forward Knee/Palm Pose, Cow Head Pose, Lion Pose, Fish Pose, Cobra Pose, Camel Pose.

Foods:

Yogatherapy Cleansing Program. Yogatherapy Diet, especially garlic, onions, cayenne, ginger, radishes, cabbage, comfrey, sprouts, leafy greens, figs, citrus fruits. Avoid dairy products until condition has cleared.

Juice Formula:

carrot 8 oz., radish 2 oz., lemon 2 oz.

Supplements:

A 10,000–25,000 i.u.

Beta-Carotene 25,000 I.U.
B-complex 50–100 mg.
C with Bioflavonoids 2–6 grams
D 400–1,000 I.U.
Calcium 1,000 mg.
High Potency Multi Mineral
N,N,Dimethylglycine (DMG) 100 mg.

Herb Teas:

Chickweed, Coltsfoot, Comfrey Leaf or Root, Elecampane, Eucalyptus, Fenugreek, Goldenseal, Hyssop, Licorice Root, Lobelia, Mullein, Red Clover, Sage, Saw Palmetto, Slippery Elm, Wood Betony.

Herbal Formulas:

#47, #56

Cold Extremities

Yoga Postures:

Soorya Namaskar, Rejuvenation Series, Triangle Pose, Standing Leg Stretch, Palm to Floor Pose, Pelvic Pose, Rock Pose, Leg Splits, *Mahamudra* 1, 2, 3.

Foods:

Yogatherapy Diet, especially nuts, seeds, whole grains, garlic, onions, cayenne, brewer's yeast.

Juice Formula:

carrot 6 oz., beet 4 oz., parsley 2 oz.

Supplements:

Niacin 100–250 mg.
C with Bioflavonoids 2–6 grams
E 400–800 I.U.
Brewer's Yeast 2 Tbsp.

Herb Teas:

Burdock Root, Comfrey Leaf or Root, Ginger, Lobelia, Yarrow.

Herbal Formulas:

#71

Colds

Yoga Postures:

The Squat, Palm Pose, One Legged Pose, Forward Knee/Palm Pose, Rock Pose, Hero Pose, Corpse Pose.

Foods:

During colds, lemon water fast. If colds are a recurring problem, Yogatherapy Cleansing Program. Then, Yogatherapy Diet, especially fresh green vegetable juices. Minimal intake of dairy products.

Juice Formula:

1 fresh lemon in hot water, with garlic 2 cloves,
OR
celery 6 oz., radish 4 oz., lemon 2 oz.

Supplements:

C with Bioflavonoids 1–2 grams every 2 hours during a cold, otherwise 2–6 grams
Beta-Carotene 25,000 I.U.
A 10,000–25,000 I.U.
Kelp 3–6 tablets
B-complex 50 mg.
Pantothenic Acid 250–1,000 mg.

Herb Teas:

Bayberry, Chickweed, Coltsfoot, Comfrey Leaf or Root, Elecampane, Eucalyptus,

Ginger, Goldenseal, Hyssop, Lobelia, Mullein, Peppermint, Sage, Sarsaparilla, Yarrow. Also cayenne and garlic in food.

Herbal Formulas:

#13–17, #47, #56, #57, #60, #69, #70

Colitis

Yoga Postures:

Soorya Namaskar, Rejuvenation Series, The Squat, Triangle Pose, Standing Leg Stretch, Inverted Leg Pose, Supine Spinal Twist, Rock Pose, *Mahamudra* 1,2,3, Abdominal Tensor Pose, Inclined Spinal Twist, Spinal Twist, Grasshopper Pose, Locust Pose, Boat Pose, Bow Pose, Cobra Pose, Bridge Pose, Plow Pose, Reverse Seal, Shoulder Stand.

Foods:

Repeated short juice fasts, Yogatherapy Cleansing Program, then Yogatherapy Diet, especially leafy greens, whole grains.

Juice Formula:

carrot 8 oz., cucumber 2 oz., beet 2 oz.

Supplements:

A 10,000–25,000 I.U.
B-complex 50–150 mg.
C with Bioflavonoids 2–6 grams
B_{12} 1,000 mcg.
N,N,Dimethylglycine (DMG) 100 mg.
High Potency Multi Mineral
Kelp 3–6 tablets
Brewer's Yeast 2 Tbsp.
Lecithin Granules 2 Tbsp.
Multiple Digestive Enzymes 1 with each meal for two months
MegaDophilus 1/4 tsp. 3 times daily

Herb Teas:

Alfalfa, Barberry, Catnip, Chamomile, Chaparral, Comfrey Leaf or Root, Ginseng, Goldenseal, Licorice Root, Parsley, Red Clover, Slippery Elm

Herbal Formulas:

#70, #74, #77

Constipation

Yoga Postures:

Soorya Namaskar, Rejuvenation Series, The Squat, Triangle Pose, Side Stretch, Knee to Chest Pose, Supine Knee to Chest Pose, Wind Eliminating Pose, Supine Spinal Twist, Pelvic Pose, Rock Pose, Inclined Spinal Twist, Grasshopper Pose, Bridge Pose, Plow Pose, Reverse Seal, Shoulder Stand.

Foods:

Yogatherapy Cleansing Program. Yogatherapy Diet, especially salads, bran, seeds, nuts, sprouted grains, sauerkraut, apples, cayenne, brewer's yeast, buttermilk, yogurt, flaxseed, psyllium seed.

Juice Formula:

apple 8 oz., spinach 4 oz.,
OR
carrot 6 oz., beet 3 oz., spinach 3 oz.

Supplements:

A 10,000–25,000 I.U.
B-complex 50–100 mg.
C with Bioflavonoids 2–6 grams
B_{12} 50 mcg.
High Potency Multi Minerals
Kelp 3 tablets with each meal
Lecithin Granules 2 Tbsp.
Brewer's Yeast 2 Tbsp.

Multiple Digestive Enzymes 1 with each meal for 2 months
MegaDophilus 1/4 tsp. 2 times daily

Herb Teas:

Barberry, Chaparral, Chickweed, Damiana, Elder, Goldenseal, Licorice Root, Mandrake, Senna.

Herbal Formulas:

#12, #35, #37, #59, #71

Cystitis

Yoga Postures:

The Squat, Wide Squat, Standing Leg Stretch, Forward Knee Pose, Forward Knee Pose with Back Stretch, Knee to Chest Pose, Seminal Control Pose, Inverted Leg Pose, Crotch Stretch, Pelvic Pose, Hero Pose, Butterfly Pose, Leg Splits, *Mahamudra* 1, 2, 3, Grasshopper Pose, Locust Pose, Reverse Seal, Shoulder Stand.

Foods:

Yogatherapy Cleansing Program, then Yogatherapy Diet, especially watermelon, pineapple, berries, leafy greens, garlic, onions, fresh green juices.

Juice Formula:

carrot 4 oz., celery 4 oz., spinach 4 oz.

Supplements:

A 10,000–25,000 I.U.
Beta-Carotene 25,000 I.U.
C with Bioflavonoids 2–6 grams
D 400–1,000 I.U.
High Potency Multi Minerals
Kelp 3–6 tablets
Alfalfa 4 tablets 3 times daily
Kyolic Liquid 1/2 tsp. 2 times daily

Herb Teas:

Agrimony, Alfalfa, Buchu, Burdock Root, Chaparral, Echinacea, Goldenrod, Goldenseal, Hops, Horsetail, Juniper Berries, Nettle, Parsley, Red Clover, Uva Ursi, Yarrow.

Herbal Formulas:

#33, #34, #75

Diabetes

Note: Diabetes is a condition which requires medical supervision. If you are diabetic and are considering employing any of the recommendations given below, consult a physician before doing so.

Yoga Postures:

Soorya Namaskar, Rejuvenation Series, Standing Back Stretch, Forward Knee Pose, Forward Knee Pose with Back Stretch, Forward Knee/Palm Pose, Celibate Pose, Pelvic Pose, *Mahamudra* 1, 2, 3, Abdominal Tensor Pose, Spinal Twist, Bow Pose, Camel Pose, Wheel Pose, Reverse Seal.

Foods:

Yogatherapy Diet, especially sea vegetables, leafy greens, whole grains, seafood, poultry, fresh vegetable juices. Avoid sweet foods, even "natural" sweets.

Juice Formula:

carrot 4 oz., spinach 4 oz., lettuce 2 oz., parsley 2 oz.

Supplements:

A 10,000–25,000 I.U.
B-complex 50–100 mg.
C with Bioflavonoids 2–6 grams
D 400–1,000 I.U.
E 400 I.U.
High Potency Multi Mineral

GTF Chromium III 200 mcg.
Kelp 3 tablets, 3 times daily
Brewer's Yeast 2 Tbsp.
Lecithin Granules 2 Tbsp.

Herb Teas:

Barberry, Bayberry, Dandelion, Fenugreek, Ginseng, Goldenseal, Parsley, Saw Palmetto, Yarrow, Yellow Dock.

Herbal Formulas:

#36, #43, #71, #76

Diarrhea

Yoga Postures:

Soorya Namaskar, Rejuvenation Series, The Squat, Triangle Pose, Standing Leg Stretch, Inverted Leg Pose, Supine Spinal Twist, Rock Pose, *Mahamudra* 1, 2, 3, Abdominal Tensor Pose, Inclined Spinal Twist, Spinal Twist, Grasshopper Pose, Locust Pose, Boat Pose, Bow Pose, Cobra Pose, Bridge Pose, Plow Pose, Reverse Seal, Shoulder Stand.

Foods:

For Recurring Diarrhea, Yogatherapy Cleansing Program. Then Yogatherapy Diet, especially apples, whole grains, raw shredded potatoes.

Juice Formula:

celery 6 oz., spinach 2 oz., lettuce 2 oz., parsley 2 oz.

Supplements:

A 10,000–25,000 I.U.
B-complex 50–100 mg.
C with Bioflavonoids 2 grams
B_{12} 500–1,000 mcg.
N,N,Dimethylglycine (DMG) 100 mg.
High Potency Multi Mineral

Kelp 3 tablets with each meal
Lecithin Granules 2 Tbsp.
Brewer's Yeast 2 Tbsp.
Multiple Digestive Enzymes 1 with each meal for two months
MegaDophilus 1/4 tsp. 3 times daily

Herb Teas:

Barberry, Bayberry, Catnip, Chamomile, Chaparral, Ginger, Goldenseal, Peppermint, Rue, Slippery Elm, Yellow Dock.

Herbal Formulas:

#70

Dysentery

Yoga Postures:

Soorya Namaskar, Rejuvenation Series, The Squat, Triangle Pose, Standing Leg Stretch, Inverted Leg Pose, Supine Spinal Twist, Rock Pose, *Mahamudra* 1, 2, 3, Abdominal Tensor Pose, Boat Pose, Bow Pose, Cobra Pose, Bridge Pose, Plow Pose, Reverse Seal, Shoulder Stand.

Foods:

Yogatherapy Cleansing Program, especially garlic, onions.

Juice Formula:

carrot 6 oz., celery 6 oz., garlic 2 cloves.

Supplements:

A 10,000–25,000 I.U.
B-complex 50–100 mg.
C with Bioflavonoids 2–6 grams
B_{12} 500–1,000 mcg.
N,N,Dimethylglycine (DMG) 100 mg.
High Potency Multi Mineral
Kelp 3 tablets

Brewer's Yeast 2 Tbsp.
Multiple Digestive Enzymes 1 with each meal for 2 months
Kyolic Liquid 1/2 tsp. 3 times daily

Herb Teas:

Alfalfa, Barberry, Burdock Root, Chaparral, Comfrey Leaf or Root, Echinacea, Fennel, Goldenrod, Goldenseal, Papaya Leaf, Peppermint, Slippery Elm, Uva Ursi, Valerian, Wormwood, Yellow Dock.

Herbal Formulas:

#44, #70

Ear Trouble (congestion, infection)

Yoga Postures:

Palm Pose, Neck Pose, Forward Knee/Palm Pose, Lion Pose, Wheel Pose, Plow Pose, Reverse Seal, Shoulder Stand.

Foods:

Yogatherapy Cleansing Program. Yogatherapy Diet, especially raw garlic, onions, fresh hot chilis. Eliminate dairy products in cases of congestion and infection until well.

Juice Formula:

celery 6 oz., radish 4 oz., lemon 2 oz.

Supplements:

A 10,000–25,000 I.U.
Beta-Carotene 25,000 I.U.
B-complex 50 mg.
Niacin 50 mg.
D 400 I.U.
High Potency Multi Mineral
Calcium 1,000 mg.
Kyolic Liquid 1/2 tsp. 2 times daily
C with Bioflavonoids 2–6 grams

Herbs Teas:

Chaparral, Chickweed, Coltsfoot, Comfrey Leaf or Root, Echinacea, Eucalyptus, Goldenseal, Hyssop, Lobelia, Mullein, Red Clover, Sage.

Herbal Formulas:

#20, #70

Eczema

Yoga Postures:

Soorya Namaskar, Rejuvenation Series, Triangle Pose, Side Stretch, Standing Leg Stretch, Forward Knee Pose, Forward Knee/Palm Pose, Moving Knee to Chest Pose, Pelvic Pose, Rock Pose, Lotus Pose, *Mahamudra* 1, 2, 3, Peacock Pose, Plow Pose, Reverse Seal, Shoulder Stand.

Foods:

Yogatherapy Diet, especially fresh green juices, leafy greens, whole grains, nuts, and seeds.

Juice Formula:

celery 4 oz., spinach 4 oz., lettuce 2 oz., parsley 2 oz.

Supplements:

A 10,000–25,000 I.U.
Beta-Carotene 25,000 I.U.
D 400–1,000 I.U.
C with Bioflavonoids 2–6 grams
B-complex 50–100 mg.
High Potency Multi Mineral
Kelp 3–6 tablets
Zinc 25–50 mg.
Alfalfa 3 tablets with each meal
Niacin 50 mg.

Herb Teas:

Alfalfa, Bayberry, Burdock Root, Chaparral, Comfrey Leaf or Root, Elecampane, Goldenseal, Horsetail, Hyssop, Parsley, Red Clover, Sarsaparilla, Sassafras, Yellow Dock.

Herbal Formulas:

#7, #10, #48, #70

Eyes (dimming of vision)

Yoga Postures:

Standing Leg Stretch, Palm to Floor Pose, *Mahamudra* 1, 2, 3, Fish Pose, Wheel Pose, Plow Pose, Reverse Seal, Shoulder Stand.

Foods:

Yogatherapy Diet, especially foods high in vitamin A.

Juice Formula:

carrot 10 oz., parsley 2 oz.

Supplements:

A 10,000–25,000 I.U.
B-complex 50 mg.
B_2 100 mg.
Niacin 50 mg.
C with Bioflavonoids 2 grams
E 400 I.U.
Kelp 3 tablets
High Potency Multi Mineral

Herb Teas:

Alfalfa, Burdock Root, Comfrey Leaf or Root, Eyebright, Horsetail, Parsley, Rue.

Herbal Formulas:

#22

Fatigue

Yoga Postures:

Soorya Namaskar, Rejuvenation Series, *Mahamudra* 1, 2, 3, Locust Pose, Boat Pose, Bow Pose, Cobra Pose, Bridge Pose, Camel Pose, Wheel Pose, Plow Pose, Reverse Seal, Shoulder Stand.

Foods:

Yogatherapy Diet, especially fresh vegetable juices, brewer's yeast, ginger, sprouts, nuts and seeds.

Juice Formula:

carrot 6 oz., beet 4 oz., parsley 2 oz.

Supplements:

A 10,000–25,000 I.U.
C with Bioflavonoids 2–6 grams
E 400 I.U.
B-complex 50–100 mg.
High Potency Multi Minerals
Brewer's Yeast 2 Tbsp.
Lecithin Granules 2 Tbsp.
Kelp 3–6 tablets
Kyolic Liquid 1/2 tsp.
N,N,Dimethylglycine (DMG) 100 mg.
Octacosanol 375–5,000 mcg.
Bee Pollen 1/2 tsp.

Herb Teas:

Ginger, Ginseng, Gotu Kola, Lobelia, Saw Palmetto. Also, chia seed, cayenne, and garlic in food.

Herbal Formulas:

#21, #23, #62–66, #68, #69, #71, #72, #74, #76, #78

Halitosis

Yoga Postures:

Knee to Chest Pose, Supine Knee to Chest Pose, Wind Eliminating Pose, Supine Spinal Twist, Pelvic Pose, Rock Pose, *Mahamudra* 1, 2, 3, Peacock Pose.

Foods:

Yogatherapy Cleansing Program. Yogatherapy Diet, especially green vegetables, brewer's yeast, papaya, parsley, comfrey, yogurt, kefir.

Juice Formula:

carrot 6 oz., spinach 4 oz., parsley 2 oz.

Supplements:

C with Bioflavonoids 2–6 grams
B-complex 50 mg.
Brewer's Yeast 2 Tbsp.
Kelp 3–6 tablets
Alfalfa 6 tablets
Multiple Digestive Enzymes 1 with each meal for 2 months
MegaDophilus 1/4 tsp. 2 times daily

Herb Teas:

Alfalfa, Barberry, Bayberry, Buchu, Chaparral, Comfrey Leaf or Root, Echinacea, Fennel, Goldenrod, Goldenseal, Hyssop, Lobelia, Papaya Leaf, Parsley, Peppermint, Senna, Yarrow.

Herbal Formulas:

#18, #19, #71

Headaches

Yoga Postures:

The Squat, Triangle Pose, Standing Leg Stretch, Palm to Floor Pose, Forward Knee/Palm Pose, Pelvic Pose, Lotus Spinal Stretch, Wheel Pose, Plow Pose, Reverse Seal, Shoulder Stand.

Foods:

Yogatherapy Diet, especially fresh green juices.

Juice Formula:

carrot 6 oz., spinach 4 oz., parsley 2 oz.

Supplements:

B-complex 50 mg.
C with Bioflavonoids 2–4 grams
Niacin 50–250 mg.
Calcium 1,000 mg.
High Potency Multi Vitamin
High Potency Multi Mineral
Lecithin Granules 2 Tbsp.

Herb Teas:

Black Cohosh, Catnip, Chamomile, Hops, Lobelia, Passion Flower, Saint-John's-Wort, Skullcap, Valerian, Wood Betony.

Herbal Formulas:

#41, #42, #77

Heart Disease

Yoga Postures:

Palm Pose, One Legged Pose, Triangle Pose, Side Stretch, Standing Back Stretch, Forward Knee Pose with Back Stretch, Forward Knee/Palm Pose, Pointing Pose, Cow Head Pose, Lotus Spinal Stretch.

Foods:

Yogatherapy Cleansing Program, Yogatherapy Diet, especially leafy greens, sprouts, cooked whole grains, fresh seeds and nuts, pears.

Juice Formula:

carrot 6 oz., beet 2 oz., celery 4 oz.

Supplements:

A 10,000–25,000 i.u.
B-complex 50 mg.
E 400–800 i.u.
High Potency Multi Mineral
Calcium 1,000 mg.
Magnesium 500 mg.
Lecithin Granules 2 Tbsp.
Niacin 50–250 mg.
Kelp 3–6 tablets
Kyolic Liquid 1/2 tsp. 2 times daily

Herb Teas:

Alfalfa, Hawthorn Berries, Lobelia

Herbal Formulas:

#28, #71, #75, #76

Hemorrhoids

Yoga Postures:

The Squat, Wide Squat, Forward Knee Pose, Supine Knee to Chest Pose, Celibate Pose, Pelvic Pose, Rock Pose, Hero Pose, Bridge Pose, Plow Pose, Reverse Seal, Shoulder Stand.

Foods:

Yogatherapy Cleansing Program. Yogatherapy Diet, especially fresh green vegetables, buttermilk, yogurt.

Juice Formula:

carrot 6 oz., spinach 4 oz., parsley 2 oz.

Supplements:

A 10,000–25,000 I.U.
B-complex 50 mg.
E 400 I.U.
C with Bioflavonoids 2–4 grams
Kelp 3–6 tablets

Herb Teas:

Barberry, Bayberry, Burdock Root, Chaparral, Comfrey Leaf or Root, Echinacea, Goldenseal, Mullein, Nettle, Stone Root. Also, cayenne in food.

Herbal Formulas:

#70, #71

Hernia

Yoga Postures:

Celibate Pose, Pelvic Pose, Rock Pose, Hero Pose, Lotus Pose, Bridge Pose, Wheel Pose, Plow Pose, Reverse Seal, Shoulder Stand.

Foods:

Yogatherapy Diet, especially all high fiber foods.

Juice Formula:

celery 4 oz., spinach 4 oz., lettuce 2 oz., parsley 2 oz.

Supplements:

High Potency Multi Mineral
High Potency Multi Vitamin
Kelp 3–6 tablets
C with Bioflavonoids 2–4 grams
E 400 I.U.

Herb Teas:

Comfrey Leaf or Root, Horsetail

Herbal Formulas:

#11

Hypoglycemia

Yoga Postures:

Soorya Namaskar, Rejuvenation Series, Standing Back Stretch, Forward Knee Pose, Forward Knee Pose with Back Stretch, Forward Knee/Palm Pose, Celibate Pose, Pelvic Pose, *Mahamudra* 1, 2, 3, Abdominal Tensor Pose, Spinal Twist, Bow Pose, Camel Pose, Wheel Pose, Reverse Seal.

Foods:

Yogatherapy Diet, especially sea vegetables, leafy greens, whole grains, raw milk, yogurt, brewer's yeast, seafood. Avoid sweet foods, even "natural" sweets.

Juice Formula:

carrot 4 oz., spinach 4 oz., lettuce 2 oz., parsley 2 oz.

Supplements:

A 10,000–25,000 I.U.
B-complex 50–100 mg.
C with Bioflavonoids 2–6 grams
D 400–1,000 I.U.
E 400 I.U.

High Potency Multi Mineral
Kelp 3-6 tablets
Brewer's Yeast 2 Tbsp.
Lecithin Granules 2 Tbsp.
GTF Chromium III 200 mcg.

Herb Teas:

Barberry, Bayberry, Dandelion, Fenugreek, Ginger, Goldenseal, Yellow Dock.

Herbal Formulas:

#30, #36, #71

Indigestion

Yoga Postures:

Soorya Namaskar, Rejuvenation Series, The Squat, Triangle Pose, Side Stretch, Standing Leg Stretch, Standing Back Stretch, Knee to Chest Pose, Supine Knee to Chest Pose, Supine Spinal Twist, Rock Pose, *Mahamudra* 1, 2, 3, Inclined Spinal Twist, Spinal Twist, Boat Pose, Bow Pose, Cobra Pose, Peacock Pose, Bridge Pose.

Foods:

Yogatherapy Cleansing Program. Yogatherapy Diet, especially papaya, apples, pineapple, watermelon, comfrey, figs, ripe tomatoes. Eat simple combinations of foods at a meal. Leafy greens, raw or steamed, sauerkraut, garlic, whole cooked grains, yogurt, kefir, buttermilk, brewer's yeast, mint, ginger.

Juice Formula:

pineapple 12 oz.,
OR
pineapple 8 oz., ginger 1 oz.,
OR
celery 6 oz., spinach 4 oz., parsley 2 oz.

Supplements:

Papaya Enzymes 1 tablet with each meal
Multiple Digestive Enzymes 1 tablet with each meal for two months

Kelp 3 tablets with each meal
Alfalfa 3 tablets with each meal
High Potency Multi Vitamin
High Potency Multi Mineral
MegaDophilus 1/4 tsp. 2 times daily

Herb Teas:

Alfalfa, Bayberry, Chamomile, Chaparral, Comfrey Leaf or Root, Echinacea, Elecampane, Eucalyptus, Ginger, Juniper Berries, Nettle, Papaya Leaf, Peppermint, Virginia Snakeroot, Wormwood, Yellow Dock.

Herbal Formulas:

#18, #19, #71, #76

Influenza

Yoga Postures:

Any postures you can comfortably perform, to keep the body somewhat flexible, especially *Mahamudra* 1, 2, 3, and Corpse Pose.

Foods:

Lemon Water Fast until well. Yogatherapy Cleansing Diet, especially citrus fruits, fresh juices.

Juice Formula:

celery 6 oz., radish 4 oz., lemon 2 oz.

Supplements:

C with Bioflavonoids 1–2 grams every 2 hours during flu
Pantothenic Acid 250–1,000 mg.
B-complex 50 mg.
Kyolic Liquid 1/2 tsp. 3 times daily

Herb Teas:

Bayberry, Chickweed, Coltsfoot, Comfrey Leaf or Root, Echinacea, Elecampane,

Eucalyptus, Ginger, Ginseng, Goldenseal, Hyssop, Lobelia, Mullein, Sarsaparilla, Yarrow, Yellow Dock.

Herbal Formulas:

#13–17, #56, #57, #60, #62, #69–71

Insomnia

Yoga Postures:

Soorya Namaskar, Rejuvenation Series, The Squat, Easy Pose, Rock Pose, Hero Pose, Lotus Pose, *Mahamudra* 1, 2, 3, Plow Pose, Reverse Seal, Shoulder Stand, Corpse Pose.

Foods:

Yogatherapy Diet.

Juice Formula:

celery 4 oz., spinach 4 oz., lettuce 2 oz., parsley 2 oz.

Supplements:

Calcium 1,000 mg.
C with Bioflavonoids 2–4 grams
B-complex 50 mg.
Brewer's Yeast 2 Tbsp.
Kelp 3–6 tablets
A 10,000 i.u.
E 400 i.u.
High Potency Multi Mineral
Tryptophan 500 mg. 20 minutes before bedtime

Herb Teas:

Catnip, Chamomile, Hops, Passionflower, Skullcap, Valerian.

Herbal Formulas:

#4, #77

Kidney Disorders

Yoga Postures:

Soorya Namaskar, Rejuvenation Series, The Squat, Triangle Pose, Side Stretch, Standing Back Stretch, Forward Knee Pose with Back Stretch, Moving Knee to Chest Pose, Inverted Leg Pose, Supine Spinal Twist, Pelvic Pose, Inclined Spinal Twist, Spinal Twist, Fish Pose, Grasshopper Pose, Locust Pose, Boat Pose, Bow Pose, Cobra Pose, Bridge Pose, Camel Pose, Wheel Pose, Plow Pose, Reverse Seal, Shoulder Stand.

Foods:

Yogatherapy Cleansing Program. Yogatherapy Diet, especially celery, parsley, cucumbers, leafy greens, garlic, watermelon.

Juice Formula:

carrot 4 oz., celery 4 oz., spinach 4 oz.

Supplements:

A 10,000–25,000 I.U.
B-complex 50 mg.
C with Bioflavonoids 2–6 grams
E 400 I.U.
Kelp 3–6 tablets

Herb Teas:

Alfalfa, Buchu, Burdock Root, Chaparral, Elder, Elecampane, Goldenrod, Goldenseal, Hawthorn Berries, Juniper Berries, Licorice Root, Parsley, Squaw Vine, Uva Ursi, Wood Betony, Yarrow.

Herbal Formulas:

#33, #34, #71, #75

Liver, Gallbladder Disorders

Yoga Postures:

Soorya Namaskar, Rejuvenation Series, Triangle Pose, Standing Leg Stretch, Palm to Floor Pose, Knee to Chest Pose, Supine Knee to Chest Pose, Wind Eliminating Pose, Moving Knees to Chest Pose, Supine Spinal Twist, *Mahamudra* 1, 2, 3, Inclined Spinal Twist, Spinal Twist, Boat Pose, Bow Pose, Cobra Pose, Peacock Pose, Bridge Pose, Plow Pose, Reverse Seal, Shoulder Stand.

Foods:

Yogatherapy Cleansing Program. Yogatherapy Diet, especially carrots, beets, leafy greens, radishes, raw nuts and seeds, brewer's yeast, garlic, virgin olive oil.

Juice Formula:

carrot 8 oz., beet 4 oz.,
OR
carrot 6 oz., cucumber 2 oz., beet 2 oz., parsley 2 oz.

Supplements:

A 10,000–25,000 I.U.
D 400–1,000 I.U.
E 400 I.U.
C with Bioflavonoids 2–6 grams
Lecithin Granules 2 Tbsp.
Kelp 3 tablets 3 times daily
Brewer's Yeast 2 Tbsp.
High Potency Multi Mineral
Kyolic Liquid 1/2 tsp. 2 times daily

Herb Teas:

Agrimony, Barberry, Bayberry, Chaparral, Golden Seal, Mandrake, Red Clover, Wormwood, Yarrow, Yellow Dock.

Herbal Formulas:

#36, #70

Lungs, Asthma

Yoga Postures:

Soorya Namaskar, Rejuvenation Series, Palm Pose, One Legged Pose, Neck Pose, Triangle Pose, Side Stretch, Standing Back Stretch, Forward Knee Pose, Forward Knee Pose with Back Stretch, Forward Knee/Palm Pose, Pointing Pose, Cow Head Pose, Lion Pose, Lotus Spinal Stretch, Cobra Pose, Camel Pose, Wheel Pose.

Foods:

Yogatherapy Cleansing Program, then Yogatherapy Diet, especially garlic, onions, cayenne, ginger, radishes, cabbage, comfrey, sprouts, leafy greens, figs, citrus fruits.

Juice Formula:

carrot 8 oz., radish 2 oz., lemon 2 oz.

Supplements:

A 10,000–25,000 I.U.
Beta-Carotene 25,000 I.U.
B-complex 50 mg.
C with Bioflavonoids 2–6 grams
D 400–1,000 I.U.
Calcium 1,000 mg.
High Potency Multi Mineral
N,N,Dimethylglycine (DMG) 100 mg.

Herb Teas

Chickweed, Coltsfoot, Comfrey Leaf or Root, Elecampane, Eucalyptus, Ginger, Goldenseal, Horsetail, Hyssop, Licorice Root, Lobelia, Mullein.

Herbal Formulas:

#2, #6, #17, #56

Male Impotence, Prostate Disorders

Yoga Postures:

Soorya Namaskar, Rejuvenation Series, The Squat, Wide Squat, Forward Knee Pose, Forward Knee Pose with Back Stretch, Seminal Control Pose, Celibate Pose, Crotch Stretch, Pelvic Pose, Hero Pose, Lotus Pose, Butterfly Pose, Leg Splits, *Mahamudra* 1, 2, 3, Grasshopper Pose, Locust Pose, Reverse Seal.

Foods:

Yogatherapy Diet, especially nuts, seeds, raw egg yolk, whole grains, raw goat milk, bee pollen, raw honey, brewer's yeast.

Juice Formula:

carrot 4 oz., celery 4 oz., spinach 4 oz.

Supplements:

High Potency Multi Vitamin
High Potency Multi Mineral
C with Bioflavonoids 2–6 grams
E 400 I.U.
Brewer's Yeast 2 Tbsp.
B-complex 50 mg.
Zinc 25–50 mg.
Wheat Germ Oil 1–2 tsp.
Octacosanol 375–5,000 mcg.
Kyolic Liquid 1/2 tsp. 2 times daily
N,N,Dimethylglycine (DMG) 100 mg.

Herb Teas:

For Impotence: Damiana, Ginger, Ginseng, Gotu Kola, Sarsaparilla, Saw Palmetto, Yohimbe. Also garlic in food.
For Prostate: Alfalfa, Buchu, Burdock Root, Chaparral, Goldenrod, Juniper Berries, Nettle, Parsley, Squaw Vine, Stoneroot, Uva Ursi, Wood Betony, Yarrow.

Herbal Formulas:

#21, #31, #46, #62–66, #71, #72, #76, #78

Menopause

Yoga Postures:

Soorya Namaskar, Rejuvenation Series, The Squat, Wide Squat, Pelvic Pose, Easy Pose, Rock Pose, Lotus Pose, Butterfly Pose, Leg Splits, *Mahamudra* 1, 2, 3, Spinal Twist, Grasshopper Pose, Locust Pose, Boat Pose, Bow Pose, Cobra Pose, Bridge Pose, Reverse Seal.

Foods:

Yogatherapy Diet, especially whole grains, nuts, seeds, brewer's yeast, raw goat milk, raisins, mission figs, black currants.

Juice Formula:

celery 4 oz., spinach 4 oz., lettuce 2 oz., parsley 2 oz.

Supplements:

A 10,000–25,000 I.U.
C with Bioflavonoids 2–6 grams
B-complex 50–100 mg.
Brewer's Yeast 2 Tbsp.
High Potency Multi Mineral
Kelp 3–6 tablets
Calcium 1,000–2,000 mg.
Lecithin Granules 2 Tbsp.
E 400–800 I.U.
Zinc 25 mg.
Iron 30 mg.
GLA 3 capsules

Herb Teas:

Black Cohosh, Blue Cohosh, Crampbark, Ginger, Ginseng, Juniper Berries, Passionflower, Rue, Saint-John's-Wort, Saw Palmetto.

Herbal Formulas:

#29, #63, #67, #71, #73, #75

Menstrual Disorders, PMS (cramping, edema, discomfort)

Yoga Postures:

Soorya Namaskar, Rejuvenation Series, The Squat, Wide Squat, Pelvic Pose, Easy Pose, Rock Pose, Lotus Pose, Butterfly Pose, Leg Splits, *Mahamudra* 1, 2, 3, Spinal Twist, Grasshopper Pose, Locust Pose, Boat Pose, Bow Pose, Cobra Pose, Bridge Pose, Reverse Seal.

Foods:

Yogatherapy Diet, especially nuts, seeds, whole grains, raw goat milk, raisins, mission figs, black currants.

Juice Formula:

celery 4 oz., spinach 4 oz., lettuce 2 oz., parsley 2 oz.

Supplements:

A 10,000–25,000 I.U.
C with Bioflavonoids 2–6 grams
B-complex 50–100 mg.
Brewer's Yeast 2 Tbsp.
High Potency Multi Mineral
Kelp 3–6 tablets
Calcium 1,000–2,000 mg.
Lecithin Granules 2 Tbsp.
E 400–800 I.U.
Zinc 25 mg.
Iron 30 mg.
GLA 3 capsules

Herb Teas:

Black Cohosh, Blue Cohosh, Buchu, Crampbark, Ginger, Ginseng, Juniper Berries, Mullein, Parsley, Passionflower, Pennyroyal, Rue, Saint John's Wort, Squaw Vine, Uva Ursi.

Herbal Formulas:

#39, #67, #71, #73, #75

Nervousness, Relaxation, Stress Management

Yoga Postures:

Any and all postures, especially the Rejuvenation Series, Plow Pose, Reverse Seal, Shoulder Stand, Corpse Pose.

Foods:

Yogatherapy Diet, especially brewer's yeast, fresh juices, raw vegetables.

Juice Formula:

celery 6 oz., beet 3 oz., parsley 2 oz., ginger 1 oz.

Supplements:

Calcium 1,000–2,000 mg.
C with Bioflavonoids 2–4 grams
B-complex 50–100 mg.
Brewer's Yeast 2 Tbsp.
Kelp 3 tablets
A 10,000 I.U.
E 400 I.U.
High Potency Multi Mineral

Herb Teas:

Black Cohosh, Catnip, Chamomile, Hops, Lobelia, Mistletoe, Passionflower, Skullcap, Valerian.

Herbal Formulas:

#4, #40, #71, #77

Obesity

Yoga Postures:

Soorya Namaskar, Rejuvenation Series, Triangle Pose, Side Stretch, Standing Leg Stretch, Forward Knee/Palm Pose, Pointing Pose, Inverted Leg Pose, Supine Spinal Twist, Abdominal Tensor Pose, Inclined Spinal Twist, Grasshopper Pose, Locust Pose, Boat Pose, Bow Pose, Cobra Pose, Inclined Pose.

Foods:

Yogatherapy Cleansing Program. Yogatherapy Diet, especially salads, fresh fruits, fresh juices.

Juice Formula:

Grapefruit 12 oz.,
OR
celery 8 oz., parsley 2 oz., lemon 2 oz.

Supplements:

Brewer's Yeast 2 Tbsp.
Kelp 3 tablets with each meal
B_6 250–1,000 mg.
Lecithin Granules 2 Tbsp.
Choline 500 mg.
C with Bioflavonoids 2–6 grams
High Potency Multi Mineral
B-complex 50–100 mg.
High Potency Multi Vitamin
E 400 I.U.

Herb Teas:

Alfalfa, Buchu, Burdock Root, Dandelion, Elder, Goldenrod, Hops, Horsetail, Juniper Berries, Licorice Root, Nettle, Parsley, Red Clover, Uva Ursi.

Herbal Formulas:

#53, #55

Pregnancy

Yoga Postures:

For the First Five Months: Soorya Namaskar, Rejuvenation Series, The Squat, Wide Squat, Triangle Pose, Celibate Pose, Crotch Stretch, Pelvic Pose, Easy Pose, Rock Pose, Butterfly Pose, Leg Splits, Inclined Spinal Twist, Grasshopper Pose, Locust Pose, Cobra Pose, Reverse Seal.

After Five Months: The Squat, Wide Squat, Celibate Pose, Crotch Stretch, Easy Pose, Rock Pose, Butterfly Pose.

Foods:

Yogatherapy Diet, especially whole grains, seeds, nuts, fresh fruits and vegetables, raw dairy products, brewer's yeast.

Juice Formula:

carrot 6 oz., beet 2 oz., spinach 2 oz., parsley 2 oz.

Supplements:

High Potency Multi Vitamin
High Potency Multi Mineral
B-complex 50 mg.
C with Bioflavonoids 2–4 grams
D 400–1,000 I.U.
E 400–800 I.U.
Kelp 3 tablets
Brewer's Yeast 2 Tbsp.

Herb Teas:

Alfalfa, Burdock Root, Ginger, Horsetail, Raspberry Leaf.

Herbal Formulas:

#45, #67, #73, #75

Pyorrhea

Yoga Postures:

Palm to Floor Pose, Lion Pose, Wheel Pose, Plow Pose, Reverse Seal, Shoulder Stand.

Foods:

Yogatherapy Diet, especially fresh raw vegetables, fruits, and fresh vegetable juices.

Juice Formula:

carrot 4 oz., celery 4 oz., parsley 2 oz., spinach 2 oz.

Supplements:

A 10,000–25,000 I.U.
C with Bioflavonoids 2–6 grams
D 400–1,000 I.U.
B_2 100 mg.
Kelp 3 tablets
High Potency Multi Mineral
Calcium 1,000 mg.
Magnesium 500 mg.

Herb Teas:

Barberry, Burdock Root, Comfrey Leaf or Root, Goldenseal, Horsetail.

Herbal Formulas:

#52

Rejuvenation

Yoga Postures:

All, especially *Soorya Namaskar*, Rejuvenation Series, Lotus Pose, *Mahamudra* 1,

2, 3, Fish Pose, Locust Pose, Bow Pose, Cobra Pose, Camel Pose, Wheel Pose, Plow Pose, Reverse Seal, Shoulder Stand.

Foods:

Yogatherapy Cleansing Program. Yogatherapy Diet, especially seeds, sprouts, whole grains, fresh fruits, bee pollen, brewer's yeast, garlic, ginger.

Juice Formula:

carrot 6 oz., beet 2 oz., spinach 2 oz., parsley 2 oz.

Supplements:

High Potency Multi Vitamin
High Potency Multi Mineral
B-complex 50 mg.
C with Bioflavonoids 2–4 grams
E 400 i.u.
Kelp 3 tablets
Lecithin Granules 2 Tbsp.
Brewer's Yeast 2 Tbsp.
Octacosanol 375–5,000 mcg.
N,N,Dimethylglycine (DMG) 100 mg.

Herb Teas:

Alfalfa, Chaparral, Comfrey Leaf and Root, Ginger, Ginseng, Gotu Kola, Horsetail.

Herbal Formulas:

#21, #23, #62–66, #68, #69, #71, #72, #74, #76, #78

Sciatica

Yoga Postures:

Soorya Namaskar, The Squat, Wide Squat, Triangle Pose, Standing Leg Stretch, Palm to Floor Pose, Forward Knee Pose, Knee to Chest Pose, Supine Knee to Chest Pose, Hero Pose, Lotus Pose, Butterfly Pose, Leg Splits, *Mahamudra* 1, 2, 3, Plow Pose.

Foods:

Yogatherapy Diet.

Juice Formula:

celery 6 oz., beet 3 oz., parsley 2 oz., ginger 1 oz.

Supplements:

A 10,000–25,000 I.U.
B-complex 50 mg.
B_6 100 mg.
N,N,Dimethylglycine (DMG) 100 mg.
C with Bioflavonoids 2–4 grams
E 400 I.U.
Calcium 1,000 mg.
High Potency Multi Mineral
Kelp 3–6 tablets

Herb Teas:

Black Cohosh, Catnip, Passionflower, Rue, Skullcap, Wood Betony.

Herbal Formulas:

#4, #41, #42

Scoliosis

Yoga Postures:

Soorya Namaskar, Rejuvenation Series, The Squat, Palm Pose, One Legged Pose, Triangle Pose, Side Stretch, Standing Leg Stretch, Palm to Floor Pose, Forward Knee/Palm Pose, Supine Spinal Twist, Pelvic Pose, Lotus Spinal Stretch, *Mahamudra* 1, 2, 3, Plow Pose.

Foods:

Yogatherapy Diet.

Juice Formula:

carrot 4 oz., spinach 4 oz., lettuce 2 oz., parsley 2 oz.

Supplements:

High Potency Multi Vitamin
High Potency Multi Mineral
Calcium 1,000 mg.
Magnesium 500 mg.
B-complex 50 mg.
C with Bioflavonoids 2 grams
Kelp 3 tablets
N,N,Dimethylglycine (DMG) 100 mg.
E 400 I.U.

Herb Teas:

Alfalfa, Comfrey Leaf and Root, Horsetail, Parsley.

Herbal Formulas:

#11

Sinus Disorders

Yoga Postures:

Neck Pose, Lion Pose, Fish Pose, Camel Pose, Wheel Pose.

Foods:

Yogatherapy Cleansing Program. Yogatherapy Diet, especially garlic, radishes, citrus fruits, fresh juices. Be very conservative with dairy products until condition has cleared.

Juice Formula:

celery 6 oz., spinach 3 oz., radish 3 oz.

Supplements:

A 10,000–25,000 I.U.
Beta-Carotene 25,000 I.U.
B_6 250 mg.
C with Bioflavonoids 2–6 grams.
Pantothenic Acid 250 mg.
D 400–1,000 mg.
Kelp 3–6 tablets
Calcium 1,000 mg.
High Potency Multi Mineral

Herb Teas:

Eucalyptus, Goldenseal, Hyssop, Lobelia, Mullein, Peppermint, Sage.

Herbal Formulas:

#1, #2, #56

Smoking—To Quit

Yoga Postures:

Soorya Namaskar, Rejuvenation Series, Palm Pose, One Legged Pose, Neck Pose, Triangle Pose, Standing Back Stretch, Forward Knee Pose with Back Stretch, Forward Knee/Palm Pose, Lotus Spinal Stretch, *Mahamudra* 1, 2, 3, Fish Pose, Cobra Pose, Camel Pose, Inclined Pose, Wheel Pose, Reverse Seal.

Foods:

Yogatherapy Cleansing Program. Yogatherapy Diet, especially fresh juices, fresh vegetables and fruits.

Juice Formula:

carrot 8 oz., radish 2 oz., lemon 2 oz.,
 OR
carrot 4 oz., celery 4 oz., parsley 2 oz., spinach 2 oz.

Supplements:

High Potency Multi Vitamin

High Potency Multi Mineral
B-complex 50 mg.
Beta-Carotene 25,000 I.U.
C with Bioflavonoids 2–6 grams
N,N,Dimethylglycine (DMG) 100 mg.
D 400–1,000 I.U.
E 400 I.U.
Kelp 3 tablets with each meal
Kyolic Liquid 1/2 tsp. 2 times daily
Brewer's Yeast 2 Tbsp.
Multiple Digestive Enzymes 1 with each meal for two months
Lecithin Granules 2 Tbsp.

Herb Teas:

Chaparral, Chickweed, Coltsfoot, Comfrey Leaf or Root, Elecampane, Eucalyptus, Goldenseal, Horsetail, Hyssop, Licorice Root, Lobelia, Mullein, Red Clover.

Herbal Formulas:

#6, #7, #10, #47, #56, #58, #71

Spinal Flexibility

Yoga Postures:

Soorya Namaskar, Rejuvenation Series, The Squat, Wide Squat, Neck Pose, Triangle Pose, Side Stretches, Standing Leg Stretch, Palm to Floor Pose, Standing Back Stretch, Forward Knee Pose with Back Stretch, Supine Spinal Twist, Pelvic Pose, Butterfly Pose, Leg Splits, *Mahamudra* 1, 2, 3, Inclined Spinal Twist, Spinal Twist, Fish Pose, Bow Pose, Cobra Pose, Bridge Pose, Camel Pose, Wheel Pose, Plow Pose.

Foods:

Yogatherapy Diet.

Juice Formula:

carrot 4 oz., beet 4 oz., spinach 2 oz., parsley 2 oz.

Supplements:

High Potency Multi Vitamin
High Potency Multi Mineral
Kelp 3 tablets
E 400 I.U.

Herb Teas:

Burdock Root, Comfrey Leaf or Root, Horsetail.

Herbal Formulas:

#11

Stomach Disorders (cramping, nausea, acidity)

Yoga Postures:

Soorya Namaskar, Rejuvenation Series, Triangle Pose, Standing Leg Stretch, Standing Back Stretch, Knee to Chest Pose, Supine Knee to Chest Pose, Supine Spinal Twist, Rock Pose, *Mahamudra* 1, 2, 3, Inclined Spinal Twist, Spinal Twist, Boat Pose, Bow Pose, Cobra Pose, Peacock Pose, Bridge Pose.

Foods:

Yogatherapy Cleansing Program. Yogatherapy Diet, especially papaya, apples, pineapple, watermelon, comfrey, figs, ripe tomatoes. Eat simple combinations of foods at a meal. Leafy greens, raw or steamed, sauerkraut, whole cooked grains, yogurt, kefir, buttermilk, brewer's yeast, mint, ginger.

Juice Formula:

pineapple 12 oz.,
OR
pineapple 8 oz., ginger 1 oz.,
OR
celery 6 oz., spinach 4 oz., parsley 2 oz.

Supplements:

Papaya Enzymes 1 with each meal
Multiple Digestive Enzymes 1 with each meal for two months
Kelp 3 tablets with each meal

High Potency Multi Vitamin
High Potency Multi Mineral
MegaDophilus 1/4 tsp. 2 times daily
E 400 I.U.
Brewer's Yeast 2 Tbsp.
B-complex 50 mg.

Herb Teas:

Alfalfa, Burdock Root, Chaparral, Comfrey Leaf or Root, Echinacea, Elecampane, Ginger, Goldenseal, Horsetail, Licorice Root, Papaya Leaf, Peppermint.

Herbal Formulas:

#18, #19, #51, #69, #70

Thyroid Disorders

Yoga Postures:

Soorya Namaskar, Rejuvenation Series, Neck Pose, Forward Knee/Palm Pose, Lotus Spinal Stretch, Fish Pose, Cobra Pose, Bridge Pose, Camel Pose, Wheel Pose, Plow Pose, Reverse Seal, Shoulder Stand.

Foods:

Yogatherapy Diet, especially parsley, watercress, kelp, Irish moss, romaine lettuce, turnip greens, grains, nuts and seeds.

Juice Formula:

celery 4 oz., spinach 4 oz., lettuce 2 oz., parsley 2 oz.

Supplements:

High Potency Multi Vitamin
B-complex 50 mg.
C with Bioflavonoids 2–6 grams
Kelp 3 tablets, 3 times daily
High Potency Multi Mineral
E 400 I.U.

Herb Teas:

Alfalfa, Comfrey Leaf or Root, Parsley.

Herbal Formulas:

#53

Vaginitis

Yoga Postures:

The Squat, Wide Squat, Standing Leg Stretch, Forward Knee Pose, Forward Knee Pose with Back Stretch, Knee to Chest Pose, Seminal Control Pose, Inverted Leg Pose, Crotch Stretch, Pelvic Pose, Hero Pose, Butterfly Pose, Leg Splits, *Mahamudra* 1, 2, 3, Grasshopper Pose, Locust Pose, Reverse Seal, Shoulder Stand.

Foods:

Yogatherapy Cleansing Program. Yogatherapy Diet, especially fresh green vegetables, kefir, yogurt, acidophilus, sauerkraut.

Juice Formula:

carrot 4 oz., celery 4 oz., spinach 4 oz., garlic 2 cloves.

Supplements:

A 10,000–25,000 I.U.
B-complex 50 mg.
C with Bioflavonoids 2–4 grams
E 400 I.U.
High Potency Multi Mineral
Calcium 1,000 mg.
Lecithin Granules 2 Tbsp.
Brewer's Yeast 2 Tbsp.
Kyolic Liquid 1/2 tsp. 2 times daily
MegaDophilus 1/4 tsp. 3 times daily

Herb Teas:

Chaparral, Dandelion, Echinacea, Goldenrod, Goldenseal, Lobelia, Parsley, Red

Clover, Sarsaparilla, Yarrow, Yellow Dock.

Herbal Formulas:

#7, #10, #69, #73, #75

Varicose Veins

Yoga Postures:

Inverted Leg Pose, Crotch Stretch, Plow Pose, Reverse Seal, Shoulder Stand.

Foods:

Yogatherapy Diet, especially leafy greens, green peppers, fresh fruits, nuts, seeds.

Juice Formula:

carrot 6 oz., green pepper 4 oz., parsley 2 oz.

Supplements:

A 10,000–25,000 i.u.
B-complex 50 mg.
Niacin 50–250 mg.
C with Bioflavonoids 2–6 grams
E 400–800 i.u.
Kelp 3–6 tablets
Lecithin Granules 2 Tbsp.
Rutin 100 mg.
Bioflavonoid Complex 500 mg.

Herb Teas:

Alfalfa, Comfrey Leaf or Root, Burdock Root, Horsetail.

Herbal Formulas:

#11

MEDITATION PRACTICE

Meditation is not what you think. It is beyond thought, beyond the normal occurrences of waking, sleeping, and dreaming. Yet meditation can at the same time pervade these states. Meditation is both straightforward and mysterious. It is immediately available, and is cultivated over a lifetime. It is the point between negative and positive, the razor fine margin between the known and the unknown. Meditation starts out as a technique, and becomes a state of being. It begins as an endeavor, and becomes indistinguishable from all of living. Initially it is of this world, and it leads to all other worlds. Meditation is both a path and a goal, and can transform your life into pure magic.

There are thousands of meditation techniques, from traditions of all different lands. In a myriad of forms, they all offer an opportunity to clarify the mind, expand awareness, harmonize with the subtle forces of life, and to achieve deep inner balance. There is no single technique which is superior to all others. Rather, different practices are suitable to different individuals. At the same time, there are some techniques which can benefit anyone who will work with them. Meditation is not like soup; you don't taste it on the spot and decide whether or not it is good. One must work with meditation to discover its power and its subtleties. Practice is essential. A few casual attempts at meditation will do little, but persistence will yield fabulous results.

People create wild expectations about meditation, due in part to sensational occult literature. Expectations are the bane of meditation practice, because they are merely products of an overactive imagination. This is not to say that there are no fabulous experiences to be had. In fact, the world of meditation opens up incredible vistas of energy, consciousness, and experience. But one of the keys to accessing those vistas is to abandon expectations and preconceived notions. Meditation works differently than does thought. Meditative experiences arise from the vast pool of consciousness. They are not products of ingenious, contrived scheming. Learn to meditate for the pleasure of that quiet, peaceful time. Then experiences will come, at the appropriate times. After all, what good is such an experience if you don't know what to do with it, how to use it for growth? If you simply want a thrill, go to the movies. If you want to integrate experience with understanding, then meditate.

To get the most out of meditation, try to make time for daily practice, and do not hurry. Even if you only set aside fifteen minutes to meditate, let that be a time when you are undisturbed by obligations, telephones, and distractions. You will find that if you practice on an empty stomach, your mental clarity will be easier to maintain than if you practice when you are full. After eating, blood accumulates in the abdomen, and mental alertness can be diminished.

As with Yoga practice, meditate in a comfortable place, and wear non-restrictive clothing. If you have the opportunity to practice in a natural setting such as the beach or the woods, try that. Nature has a wonderful way of facilitating meditation. This is because we humans have a strong connection to the primordial energies of Nature, as those energies are the basic stuff of which we are made.

The technique of meditation offered here is very simple. Yet it can be practiced for decades, with impressive results. While the actual practice is free from complication, you will quickly find that there is a lot to this method. Unlike many other forms, this technique uses no mantras (words or sounds), no visualizations, and no exotic mental gymnastics. Instead, this meditation guides the practitioner to the very root of consciousness in a most direct manner. Do not fool yourself into thinking that you need a more exotic technique. If you can practice this meditation fully, you can do anything.

If you are not particularly flexible, then I recommend that you start out practicing this meditation sitting upright in a chair. In time, you may find it comfortable to sit in a cross-legged position.

If possible, place yourself in full lotus position. For most people this is not possible initially. If such is the case for you, choose any other cross-legged sitting position in which you can maintain an erect posture and a straight spine.

Once you are seated, place your hands palms down upon your knees. The arms are relaxed, with the shoulders loose and at ease. Pull your chin in slightly, so that your neck is straight. The tongue is placed lightly on the roof of the mouth.

This position provides for a smooth, even energy flow. It enables you to generate and circulate energy without effort, thus facilitating meditation. In this particular practice, posture is a very important component.

Seated in the correct posture, breathe through the nose, so that your breath is long and steady. The breath is not particularly deep, but it is long and drawn out, with a steady inhalation and a steady exhalation. As you breathe, fix your attention at the root of the nose, just where the nose meets the brow. With the breath long and steady, pay attention to the feeling of the breath as it passes by the spot at the inside of the root of the nose. As you inhale, you will feel the breath flowing up through the nostrils, past the root of the nose. As you exhale, you will feel the breath flowing past the root of the nose and out through the nostrils.

The object of this meditation practice is to keep your attention focused on the root of the nose, feeling the breath as it flows by that spot on the way in and out. Thoughts will arise, and as they do, return your concentration to the breath flowing by the root of the nose. There may be some discomfort somewhere in your body, but instead of paying attention to that, return your attention to the breath flowing by the root of the nose. There may be noises or distractions around you, but simply return your attention to the breath flowing by the root of the nose. Every time there is any distraction at all, whether internal or external, return your attention to the breath flowing by the root of the nose. Do this again and again.

As you practice, you may find that initially your attention span will be short, and that you may become distracted easily. But as you continue, your attention will stay in one place longer. Gradually, you will be able to pay attention to the breath flowing by the root of the nose, without becoming distracted. This one-pointed concentration allows you the opportunity to break the habitual pattern of chattering to yourself inside. Through such concentration, you will become more and more clear minded, perceptually keen, and aware of the world around you.

When the mind is not totally preoccupied with itself, then it is able to pay attention to other things. Sight, sound, smell, touch, and taste become enhanced, as the body/mind springs alive with newly liberated energy. The process is one of continuous growth and refinement.

Meditation has no beginning or end. It spills over into daily life, and changes everything. Through regular practice of this meditation technique, you can gain access to new, exciting, and magical worlds.

References

Airola, Paavo. *Are You Confused?* Phoenix, Arizona: Health Plus Publishers, 1971.

Bieler, Henry G. *Food Is Your Best Medicine.* New York: Harcourt Brace Javanovich, 1970.

Christopher, John R. *School of Natural Healing.* Provo, Utah: Bi-World Publishing, 1976.

Culpeper, Nicholas. *Culpeper's Complete Herval.* New York: Sterling Publishing Co., 1959.

Davis, Adelle. *Let's Eat Right to Keep Fit.* New York: Harcourt Brace Javanovich, 1970.

Deal, Sheldon C. *New Life through Nutrition.* Tucson, Arizona: New Life Publishing, 1974.

Heinerman, John. *Science of Herbal Medicine.* Provo, Utah: Bi-World Publishing, 1979.

Iyangar, B. K. S. *Light on Yoga.* New York: Schocken Books, 1979.

Kloss, Jethro. *Back to Eden.* Santa Barbara, Ca.: Woodbridge Press Publishing Co, 1939.

Lust, John. *Drink Your Troubles Away.* Simi Valley, Ca.: Benedict Lust Publications, 1967.

Lust, John. *The Herb Book.* Simi Valley, Ca.: Benedict Lust Publications, 1974.

Ott, John. *Health and Light.* New York: Pocket Books, 1976.

Schwarz, Jack. *Human Energy Systems.* New York: E. P. Dutton, 1980.

Sivananda, Sri Swami. *Kundalini Yoga.* Shivandagar, India: Divine Life Society, 1980.

Walker, Norman. *Raw Vegetable Juices.* Denver, Colorado: Nutri-Books Corp., 1970.

Index

Abdominal Tensor Pose, 69
Acetylcholine, 24, 109
Acidophilus, 140
Acne, 170, 171
Adenoids, Tonsils, 171
Adenosine, 100
Agricultural Chemicals, 118
Agrimony, 148
Air, 84, 85
Alcohol, 23, 100
Alcoholism, Drug
  Addiction, 172
Alfalfa, 106, 148
Aldosterone, 96
Allergies, Hay Fever, 173
Almonds, 106
Amylase, 141
Anemia, 174
Anti-stiffness factor, 106
Appetite (poor, lack of), 175
Apples, 106
Arterial Disease, 176
Arthritis, Gout, Rheumatism, 177
Ascorbic Acid, 130, 131
Aura, 31, 32
Avocados, 106, 107
Ayurveda, 19, 20, 106, 107, 110

Baba, Herakhan, 24
Back Pain, 178
Bananas, 107
Barberry, 148
Bayberry, 148
Bee Pollen, 107
Beets, 107
Beta-Carotene, 140
Betaine HCL, 141
Bio Strath, 140
Biochemical Individuality, 120
Biofeedback, 23
Bioflavonoids, 133
Biotin, 129
Black Cohosh, 148
Bladder Disorders, 179
Blood Pressure, High, 179, 180

Blood Pressure, Low, 180, 181
Blood sugar, 24
Blue Cohosh, 148
Boat Pose, 73
Bone Meal, 140, 141
Bow Pose, 73, 74
Bran, 107
Breathing, 38, 39
  Normal breath, 38
  Long deep breath, 38, 39
Bridge Pose, 75, 76
Bromelain, 110, 141
Bronchitis, 181, 182
Brown Rice, 107
Buchu, 148
Buddha, 27
Buddhism, 25
Burdock Root, 148
Butterfly Pose, 66
Buttermilk, 108

Caffeine Products, 100
Calcium, 133
Camel Pose, 76
Catnip, 149
Cayenne, 149
Celibate Pose, 59
Chakra Chart, 34–36
Chakras, 30, 32–36
  First, 32–34
  Second, 33, 35
  Third, 33, 35
  Fourth, 33, 35
  Fifth, 32, 34, 35
  Sixth, 33, 35
  Seventh, 34, 36
Chamomile, 149
Champion Juicer, 95
Chaparral, 149
Charisma, 33
Chemical Additives, 100, 118
Chewing, 102
Chia Seed, 149
Chickweed, 149
Chilis, 108
Chocolate, 100
Choline, 130
Chromium, 137, 138

Chymotrypsin, 141
Cleansing Daily Schedule, 104, 105
Cleansing Program, 102–106
Cobra Pose, 74
Cod Liver Oil, 108
Cold Extremities, 182, 183
Colds, 183, 184
Colitis, 184, 185
Coltsfoot, 149
Comfrey Leaf and Root, 149
Constipation, 185, 186
Cooking (vitamin loss), 117
Copper, 135
Corpse Pose, 80
Cosmic Consciousness, 34
Cow Head Pose, 64
Crampbark, 149
Crotch Stretch, 61
Cyanocobalamin, 127, 128
Cystitis, 186, 187

Dairy Products and Eggs, 96, 97
Damiana, 149
Dandelion, 149
Depleted Soil, 117
Desiccated Liver, 141
DES, 98
Devil's Claw, 149
Diabetes, 187, 188
Diarrhea, 188, 189
Diazepam, 23
Digestants, 141, 142
Divinity, 26, 27
Dolomite, 142
Drugs, 101
Dysentery, 189, 190

Ear Trouble (congestion, infection), 190, 191
Easy Pose, 62
Eating, Guidelines, 101, 102
Echinacea, 149
Eczema, 191, 192
Eggs, 97
Elder, 149
Elecampane, 149

Emotion, 30
Endorphins, 23
Enlightenment, 26, 27, 29
Enzymes, 94
Eucalyptus, 149
Evening Primrose Oil, 142
Eyebright, 150
Eyes (dimming of vision), 192, 193

Fasting, 111–113
Fatigue, 193, 194
Fennel, 150
Fenugreek, 150
Fiber, 94
Fish, 98, 99
Fish Pose, 71
Flaxseed, 150
Folacin, 129
Folic Acid, 129
Food Additives, 23, 24
Forward Knee/Palm Pose, 55
Forward Knee Pose, 54
Forward Knee Pose with Back Stretch, 54
Fresh Air, 84, 85
Fresh Juices, 95
Fresh Vegetables and Fruits, 94
Fruits, 94

Gandhi, Mahatma, 24
Garlic, 108, 150
Gerson Therapy, 112
Gingerroot, 108, 150
Ginseng, 150
GLA (gamma linolenic acid), 142
Goldenrod, 150
Goldenseal, 150
Gotu Kola, 150
Grains, 97, 98
Grasshopper Pose, 72
Great Dance of Illusion, 29
Guidelines for Eating, 101, 102

Halitosis, 194
Hatha Yoga, 19, 39
Hawthorn Berries, 150
Headaches, 195
Health and Light, 83
Heart Disease, 195, 196

Hemorrhoids, 196, 197
Herbal Extracts and Tablets, 163–166
Herbal Formula/Ailment Chart, 153–162
HERBAL FORMULAS:
  # 1 Allergies, 153
  # 2 Antimucus Tincture, 153
  # 3 Antiseptic Ointment, 153
  # 4 Antispasmodic and Nerve Tincture, 153
  # 5 Arthritis, Rheumatism, 154
  # 6 Asthma Syrup, 154
  # 7 Blood Cleanser, 154
  # 8 Blood Pressure (high or low), 154
  # 9 Blood Pressure (high), 154
  #10 Blood Purification, Detoxification, 154, 155
  #11 Bone, Flesh, Cartilage Builder, 155
  #12 Bowel Function, 155
  #13 Colds, Coughs, 155
  #14 Colds, Flu, 155
  #15 Cold and Flu Syrup, 155
  #16 Cold Prevention, 155
  #17 Cough Syrup, 156
  #18 Digestive Aid, 156
  #19 Digestive Disorders, 156
  #20 Ear Tincture, 156
  #21 Energy, Endurance, Stamina, 156
  #22 Eye Disorders, 156
  #23 Fatigue, Stress, Debility, 156, 157
  #24 Fever, Flu, 157
  #25 Gland Problems, 157
  #26 Glands (swollen, infected, lymph), 157
  #27 Glandular Infections, 157
  #28 Heart, 157
  #29 Hormonal Imbalances, 157
  #30 Hypoglycemia, 158

#31 Impotence, 158
#32 Insomnia, 158
#33 Kidney and Bladder, 158
#34 Kidney Function, 158
#35 Laxative, 158
#36 Liver, Gallbladder, 158, 159
#37 Lower Bowel Tonic and Cleanser, 159
#38 Memory Aid, 159
#39 Menstrual Regulator, 159
#40 Nervous Disorders, 159
#41 Pain, Headaches, 159
#42 Pain Tincture, 159, 160
#43 Pancreas, 160
#44 Parasites, 160
#45 Pre-Natal Formula, 160
#46 Prostate, Kidney, 160
#47 Respiratory Aid, 160
#48 Skin Aid, 160, 161
#49 Skin Blemishes, 161
#50 Spring Tonic, 161
#51 Stomach Tincture, 161
#52 Teeth and Gums, 161
#53 Thyroid, 161
#54 Ulcers, 161, 162
#55 Weight Control, 162
#56 Breathe Easy Herbal Decongestant, 162
#57 Gypsy Cold Care Herb Cold Medicine, 162
#58 Smoker's Tea Smoking Deterrent, 162, 163
#59 Smooth Move Herbal Laxative, 163
#60 Throat Coat Soothes Sore Throats, 163
#61 Weightless Tea Herbal Diet Aid, 163
#62 Shiu Chu Ginseng

Extract, 164
#63 East-West Blend, 164
#64 Siberian Ginseng, 164
#65 Wild American Ginseng, 164
#66 Woodsgrown Ginseng, 164
#67 Dong Quai, 164
#68 Fo-Ti, 164
#69 Ginger, 164, 165
#70 Goldenseal, 165
#71 Dragon Brew, 165
#72 Shiu Chu Ginseng, 165
#73 Tang Kuei, 165
#74 Express, 165
#75 Women's Longevity, 165
#76 Four Ginsengs, 165
#77 Peaceful, 166
#78 Sage's Ginseng, 166
Herbal Tea Bag/Ailment Chart, 162, 163
Herbs, 146–168
    Preparation and use, 147, 148
    (Individual) Herb Chart, 148–152
Hernia, 197, 198
Hero Pose, 63
Hinduism, 25
Hitler, 28
Homogenization, 97
Honey, 108
Hops, 150
Horsetail, 150
Hot and Cold Showers, 89
Hydrotherapy, 89
Hypoglycemia, 198, 199
Hyssop, 150

Illness, Dis-ease, 31
Inclined Pose, 76, 77
Inclined Spinal Twist, 70
Indigestion, 199, 200
Influenza, 200, 201
Inositol, 130
Insomnia, 201
Inverted Leg Pose, 58, 59
Iodine, 134, 135
Iron, 135

Juice/Ailment Chart, 113, 114
Juicers, 95
Juices, 95
    How to prepare, 113
Juniper Berries, 150

Karma, 27–29
Kelp, 109
Kidney Disorders, 202
Knee to Chest Pose, 56
Kyolic, 142

Lecithin, 24, 109
Leg Splits, 66, 67
Lemon-Water Diet, 103, 104
LHRH, 23
Licorice Root, 150
Life and Energy, 29, 30
Life force, 93
Lion Pose, 64
Lipase, 141
Liver, Gallbladder Disorders, 203
L-lysine, 142
Lobelia, 151
Locust Pose, 72, 73
Lotus Pose, 65
Lotus Spinal Stretch, 65
L-tryptophan, 142
Lungs, Asthma, 204

Magnesium, 133, 134
Mahamudra #1 (The Great Yogic Seal), 67, 68
Mahamudra #2, 68
Mahamudra #3, 68
Male Impotence, Prostate Disorders, 205
Mandrake, 151
Manganese, 137
MaxEPA, 142
Maya, 29
Meditation, 24, 25, 221–225
Menopause, 206
Menstrual Disorders, PMS, 207, 208
Mind (mental energy), 30
Mind/Body Relationship, 22–25
Mistletoe, 151
Moving Knees to Chest Pose, 58
Mugwort, 151

Mullein, 151
Myrrh Gum, 151

Nadis, 30
Nature—Vite Quick Reference Chart, 138–140
Neck Pose, 50
Nervousness, Relaxation, Stress Management, 208
Nettle, 151
New physics, 28
Niacin, 126
Nutrient Measure and Conversion Chart, 123, 124
Nutrient Section explained, 122, 123
Nutritional Yeast, 109
Nuts and Seeds, 95, 96

Obesity, 209
Octacosanol, 98, 111, 142
Olive Oil, 109
One Legged Pose, 50
Ott, John, 83
Ox Bile, 141

PABA (Para-Amino-Benzoic Acid), 128
Palm Pose, 49, 50
Palm to Floor Pose, 53
Pancreatin, 141
Pantothenic Acid, 128
Papain, 109, 142
Papaya, 109
Papaya Leaf, 151
Parsley, 151
Passion Flower, 151
Pasteurization, 96, 97
Patanjali, 27
Peacock Pose, 74, 75
Pelvic Pose, 62
Pennyroyal, 151
Peppermint, 151
Pepsin, 142
Pheromones, 23
Phosphatidylcholine, 24, 109
Phosphorous, 134
Phylloquinone, 132
Physical energy, 30
Physician's Desk Reference, 101
Pineapple, 110
Plow Pose, 78

232/INDEX

Pointing Pose, 55, 56
Poor Dietary Intake, 117
Potassium, 136, 137
Pralaya, 88
Prana, 38
Pregnancy, 210
Preservatives, 100
Processing and Vitamin Loss, 117
Prostaglandins, 96
Psyllium Seed, 151
Pure Water, 85–87
Pyorrhea, 211
Pyridoxine, 127

Raspberry Leaf, 151
Raw Milk, 95, 97
Raw Vegetables, 94
RDA = Recommended Dietary Allowances, 119–121
   Chart, 121
Red Clover, 151
Regularity in Schedule and Habits, 90
Reincarnation, 26
Rejuvenation, 211, 212
Rejuvenation Series, 42–48
Retinol, 124, 125
Reverse Seal, 78, 79
Riboflavin, 126
Rock Pose, 63
Rose Hips, 151
Royal Jelly, 143
Rue, 151
Runner's high, 23

Sage, 152
Saint-John's-Wort, 152
Sanskrit, 19, 29
Sarsaparilla, 152
Sassafras, 152
Saw Palmetto, 152
Sciatica, 212, 213
Scoliosis, 213, 214
Selenium, 137
Seminal Control Pose, 56, 57
Senna, 152
Sesame, 110
Sexual energy, 33
Sexual orgasm, 33
Shoulder Stand, 79, 80
Showers, 89
Side Stretch, 52

Sinus Disorders, 214, 215
Siva, 27
Skullcap, 152
Sleep, 88, 89
Sleeping on left and right sides, 88
Slippery Elm, 152
Smoking, 101
Smoking—To Quit, 215, 216
Sodium, 136
Soorya Namaskar—Salute to the Sun, 39–42
Souls, 26
Spinal Flexibility, 216, 217
Spinal Twist, 70, 71
Spirit, 30
Spirulina, 143
Sprout Chart, 110
Squat, 48, 49
Squaw Vine, 152
Standing Leg Stretch, 52
Stigmasterol, 106
Stomach Disorders, 217, 218
Stoneroot, 152
Stresses, 118
Sugars, 99
Sunshine, 83, 84
Super Foods, 106–111
Supine Knee to Chest Pose, 57
Supine Spinal Twist, 60
Survival, 33
Sushi/Sashimi, 110

Theobromine, 100
Thiamine, 125
Third Eye, 34
Thyroid Disorders, 218, 219
Transit Time and Storage, 117
Triangle Pose, 51
Trypsin, 141

Union, 25–27
Unsaturated Fatty Acids, 132
Uva Ursi, 152

Vaginitis, 219, 220
Valerian, 152
Varicose Veins, 220
Vegetables, 94
Virginia Snakeroot, 152
Vitamin A, 108, 124, 125
Vitamin B_1, 125

Vitamin B_2, 126
Vitamin B_6, 127
Vitamin B_{12}, 127, 128
Vitamin C, 130, 131
Vitamin D, 108, 131
Vitamin E, 131, 132
"Vitamin F", 132
Vitamin K, 132
Vitamin P, 133
Vital Foods, 93–99
Vitality, 30
Vitality Body, 30

Walking, 87
Water, 85–87
Way of Yoga, 25
Wheat Germ, 111
Wheat Germ Oil, 111
Wheel Pose, 77, 78
White Flour, 99, 100
Whole Grains, 97, 98
Wide Squat, 49
Will, 33
Wind Eliminating Pose, 57
Wisdom Eye, 34
Wood Betony, 152
Wormwood, 152

Yarrow, 152
Yellow Dock, 152
Yoga, 19–21, 89, 90, 98
   Definition of, 25
Yoga Postures and Exercises, 39–80
Yogatherapy, 19–22, 24–26, 31, 32, 38, 39, 84–88, 90, 95, 98, 117
   Cleansing Program, 103–106
   and Diet, 93–102
   Repertory, 168–220
Yogatherapy, Advice on Practice, 37
Yogatherapy, Contraindications, 37
Yogatherapy, Daily Plan, 36
Yogic Philosophy, 26–29
Yogis, 22, 24, 31, 83, 85, 86
Yogurt, 111
Yohimbe, 152

Zell Oxygen, 143
Zinc, 136